Pharmacology

Michael D Randall
Associate Professor and Reader in Cardiovascular Pharmacology,
School of Biomedical Sciences,
University of Nottingham Medical School, UK

Stephen PH Alexander
Associate Professor in Molecular Pharmacology,
School of Biomedical Sciences,
University of Nottingham Medical School, UK

and

David A Kendall
Professor of Pharmacology,
School of Biomedical Sciences,
University of Nottingham Medical School, UK

Pharmaceutical Press
London • Chicago

Published by the Pharmaceutical Press
An imprint of RPS Publishing
1 Lambeth High Street, London SE1 7JN, UK
100 South Atkinson Road, Suite 200, Grayslake, IL 60030-7820, USA

(**P.P**) is a trade mark of RPS Publishing
RPS Publishing is the publishing organisation of the Royal Pharmaceutical
Society of Great Britain

First published 2009

Typeset by J&L Composition, Scarborough, North Yorkshire
Printed in Great Britain by by TJ International, Padstow, Cornwall

ISBN 978 0 85369 824 1

A catalogue record for this book is available from the British Library.

Contents

Introduction to the
FASTtrack series

FASTtrack is a new series of revision guides created for undergraduate pharmacy students. The books are intended to be used in conjunction with textbooks and reference books as an aid to revision to help guide students through their exams. They provide essential information required in each particular subject area. The books will also be useful for pre-registration trainees preparing for the Royal Pharmaceutical Society of Great Britain's (RPSGB's) registration examination, and to practising pharmacists as a quick reference text.

The content of each title focuses on what pharmacy students really need to know in order to pass exams. Features include*:
- concise bulleted information
- key points
- tips for the student
- multiple choice questions (MCQs) and worked examples
- case studies
- simple diagrams.

The titles in the *FASTtrack* series reflect the full spectrum of modules for the undergraduate pharmacy degree.

Titles include:
Complementary and Alternative Medicine
Managing Symptoms in the Pharmacy
Pharmaceutical Compounding and Dispensing
Pharmaceutics: Dosage Form and Design
Pharmaceutics: Drug Delivery and Targeting
Pharmacology
Physical Pharmacy (based on Florence & Attwood's *Physicochemical Principles of Pharmacy*)
Therapeutics

There is also an accompanying website which includes extra MCQs, further title information and sample content: www.fasttrackpharmacy.com.

If you have any feedback regarding this series, please contact us at feedback@fasttrackpharmacy.com.

*Note: not all features are in every title in the series.

About the authors

Dr MICHAEL RANDALL is an Associate Professor and Reader in Cardiovascular Pharmacology; Dr STEPHEN ALEXANDER is an Associate Professor in Molecular Pharmacology; Professor DAVID KENDALL is Professor of Pharmacology. All of the authors are from the School of Biomedical Sciences, University of Nottingham, where they all teach pharmacology on the pharmacy and medical courses.

Preface

Pharmacology is a core subject within pharmacy and medicine and is the science behind the therapeutic use of drugs. A thorough knowledge of pharmacology underpins the safe and appropriate use of medicines. In understanding how a drug acts one can then anticipate its desired and, indeed, its undesired effects. Therefore, one aim of this book is to provide a brief account of drug action, as either a study or revision aid. In doing this, we have generally taken a therapeutic area and considered the major classes of drugs, their actions and, to a limited degree, their uses. Pharmacology is not about learning vast lists of drugs but it is more important to understand how key classes of drugs act.

There are many excellent brief guides to pharmacology and so our second aim was to present a study guide which deals with molecular pharmacology at a more advanced level, as this underpins the science of pharmacology. In taking this approach we believe that we have produced a book which will also be useful for advanced pharmacology studied in the later years of pharmacy and science degrees. Therefore, we believe that we have produced a study guide which should be useful at each level of undergraduate study.

The early chapters concentrate on the molecular targets of drug action and this leads in to major therapeutic areas. In these latter chapters the focus is on mechanisms of drug action rather than the disease or its treatment. Most chapters contain summary key points and self-tests. We have used a variety of approaches to self-tests. Exam formats vary between courses and so exposure to different modes should help with testing of knowledge rather than train a strategic approach to exam questions.

This study guide is meant to aid an understanding of pharmacology and should be used in conjunction with lecture material and standard textbooks of pharmacology. The knowledge gained then feeds into the study of clinical pharmacology.

Michael Randall, Stephen Alexander
and David Kendall, May 2009

chapter 1
Pharmacodynamics

Pharmacodynamics is the consideration of the targets of drug action. Of course, this depends on what constitutes a drug. Although other refinements of this definition exist, for the purposes of this book, any agent, other than a nutrient, which alters bodily functions can be considered to be a drug. In general, the targets of drugs can be divided into two types, classed either as non-specific or specific.

Non-specific targets are most often small molecules. Therapeutic responses generated through non-specific targets exploit chemistry and/or physics to achieve a desirable effect and are entirely dependent on the biodistribution of the drug.

Non-specific medicinal drug actions include:

- Antacids:
  - HCO_3^- and OH^- salts used to alleviate dyspepsia and heartburn and to neutralise acid in the stomach
- Laxatives:
  - lactulose, used to treat constipation; it acts in the lower bowel to increase osmotic pressure, retain water and accelerate softer bowel motions
- Diuretics:
  - mannitol, used to treat cerebral oedema; it acts in the kidney to increase osmotic pressure, retain water in urine and increase urinary volume
- Heavy-metal chelators:
  - desferrioxamine, used to treat iron poisoning; it chelates and absorbs iron in the gut.

Specific targets for drug action are usually macromolecules. Therapeutic responses evoked through specific targets exploit both chemistry and biology and are only partly dependent on the biodistribution of the drug. Examples of specific targets include:

- transporters (numerous)
- enzymes (numerous)
- ion channels (numerous)
- receptors (very many)
- structural proteins (very few)
- hormones (few).

The strategy for development of drugs for transporters, enzymes and receptors in classical pharmacology was based on chemically modifying the endogenous substrate or ligand to reduce metabolism and enhance affinity. Of these targets, the receptors are an exceptional class in that drugs are able to enhance (agonists) or inhibit (antagonists) the activity of the target. In contrast, the majority of drugs exploiting other drug targets are inhibitors.

Since the ion channels and transporters and receptors are dealt with in individual chapters, the remainder of this chapter deals with the remaining specific targets.

Enzymes

It is possible to divide the enzymes into two major groups, dependent on their subcellular location.

- Agents which alter intracellular enzyme activity require access to the inside of the cell, while extracellular enzyme activity can be influenced by agents which do not need to penetrate the cell membrane.
- Drugs which influence enzyme activity tend to be inhibitors which 'kill' the enzyme. They are usually derived initially from natural substrate, with suitable chemical modification to resist metabolism.
- Enzyme inhibitors lead to increased accumulation of substrate and decreased accumulation of product, either of which may produce the desired therapeutic effect (Figure 1.1).
- A rare example of a drug which acts to enhance enzyme activity is metformin, used in the treatment of type 2 diabetes mellitus. This agent acts in an undefined manner to enhance the activity of adenosine monophosphate (AMP)-activated protein kinase, thereby decreasing liver glucose production and increasing peripheral glucose uptake.
- Alternatively, enzyme activity can be harnessed for activation of drugs by metabolising a prodrug (Figure 1.1). For example, enalapril, used in the treatment of hypertension, is converted in the liver to enalaprilat, an angiotensin-converting enzyme inhibitor.

Figure 1.1 Enzymes as drug targets. (a) Under normal circumstances, enzymes catalyse the conversion of a substrate to a product. (b) The predominant influence of drugs on enzyme activity is as inhibitors, which prevent product formation or increase substrate accumulation, either of which may prove beneficial. (c) A further involvement of enzymes in drug action is where the active entity is only produced following enzymatic metabolism of a prodrug.

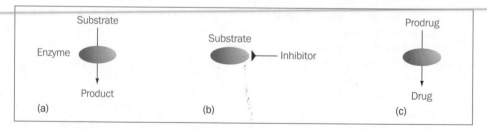

Inhibitors of extracellular enzymes

Inhibitors of extracellular enzymes regulate the extracellular environment through the accumulation of substrate and reduction of product; drugs can be charged and water-soluble.

- Neostigmine is used to treat myasthenia gravis, where autoantibodies inactivate nicotinic acetylcholine receptors at the neuromuscular junctions. It acts as an acetylcholinesterase inhibitor to increase endogenous levels of acetylcholine, thereby enhancing transmission at the skeletal neuromuscular junction.
- Tetrahydrolipstatin (orlistat) is used to treat obesity. It is an inhibitor of pancreatic lipase in the lumen of the small intestine, thereby reducing the availability of fatty acids for absorption. Not only does this result in a reduced accumulation of fats in the body, but it means that the lipid remaining in the gut acts as an osmotic laxative, resulting in steatorrhoea (fatty stools).
- Acarbose is used to treat type 2 diabetes. It is an inhibitor of disaccharidases in the mucosa of the small intestine to slow the metabolism and hence uptake of sugars following a meal, thereby reducing the peak of glucose levels in plasma.

Inhibitors of intracellular enzymes

Inhibitors of intracellular enzymes regulate the internal environment of the cell and may enter the cell, either as surrogate substrates for transporters or through being sufficiently hydrophobic so as to pass through the cell membranes.

- 5-Fluorouracil is used to treat colorectal and pancreatic cancers; it is taken up through nucleoside transporters and acts as a surrogate nucleoside for nucleic acid formation.
- Anastrozole is used to treat hormone-sensitive breast cancer in postmenopausal women; it acts as an aromatase inhibitor (see Chapter 32), thereby preventing the formation of oestrone and oestradiol, which enhance the proliferation of some types of breast cancer.
- Sildenafil is used to treat male sexual dysfunction; it functions to inhibit intracellular phosphodiesterase 5, which hydrolyses cyclic guanosine monophosphate (cGMP). Elevating cGMP in the vascular smooth muscle leads to vasorelaxation. In the corpus cavernosum of the penis, this vasorelaxation prevents blood draining from the penis, thereby engorging and stiffening it.

Suicide substrates and irreversible inhibitors

These agents act as substrates for enzymatic activity, but in the process bind irreversibly, hence the appellation of suicide.

- Eflornithine (difluoromethylornithine) is used as a cream in the treatment of female hirsutism to remove excessive facial hair, as well as an antiparasitic in the treatment of sleeping sickness. It accumulates in cells, acting as a surrogate substrate for amino acid transporters. Once in the cell, it acts as an irreversible inhibitor of ornithine decarboxylase, preventing the formation of the polyamine spermine, which has an important role in the regulation of nucleic acid replication and cell division.
- Penicillin, a β-lactam antibiotic, acts to inhibit bacterial proliferation by binding irreversibly to a transpeptidase, which cross-links peptidoglycans in the bacterial cell wall.

- Azidothymidine (AZT), used in the treatment of human immunodeficiency virus (HIV)/acquired immunodeficiency syndrome (AIDS), acts to inhibit reverse transcriptase. This enzyme is vital for replication as it functions to make a DNA copy of the viral RNA, needed for insertion into the host cell's DNA. AZT accumulates in the cell through the action of nucleoside transporters, where it is used to synthesise an azido analogue of thymidine 5'-triphosphate. This is the active entity that irreversibly inhibits reverse transcriptase. As other DNA polymerases in the cell, particularly in the mitochondria, are also less potent targets, AZT treatment is associated with cardiac damage.

Structural proteins

There are relatively few drugs which regulate structural protein function; they are mostly associated with the treatment of cancer (Chapter 32).
- Tubulin, a protein that makes up the cytoskeletal element microtubules, is the target for the anticancer drugs taxol, vinblastine, vincristine, colchicine and griseofulvin (which also has antifungal activity).

Hormones

- In the case of endocrine insufficiency, it is usually feasible simply to replace the hormone.
- If there is an excess of the hormone, normally an antagonist is used to prevent overstimulation of the receptor.
- For cytokines, however, no antagonists are yet available and so an alternative therapeutic alternative is to produce antibodies which chelate the hormone and prevent its action (see Chapter 34).

KeyPoints

- Drug specificity is determined by the ability to interact with particular target sites in the body.
- Many (or even most) therapeutic drugs act at multiple sites in the body, eliciting effects which may be beneficial or not.

chapter 2
Receptors

Receptors are the most clinically exploited group of drug targets, partly because of the opportunity to make use of receptor function in both positive and negative directions, using agonists and antagonists.

The archetypal receptor is made up of four components or domains:
1. a ligand recognition site (for nuclear receptors, often referred to as the ligand binding domain or LBD)
2. structural domain/s
3. a functional signalling domain, which performs the work of the receptor
4. regulatory domains, at which small molecules other than the orthodox ligand act to regulate receptor function (Figure 2.1).

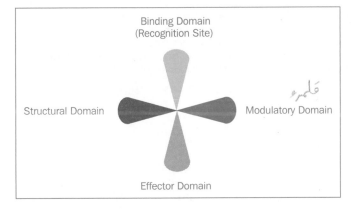

Figure 2.1 The prototypical receptor is made up of four domains, which may be physically distinct or conjoined entities.

Superfamilies of receptors

There are four superfamilies of receptors, which have many features that distinguish them in physical and biochemical terms (Table 2.1).

Each of these superfamilies is discussed below, using representative examples of the class.

7-Transmembrane domain receptors (7TMR)

7TMR, often referred to as G-protein-coupled, heptahelical or metabotropic receptors, are defined by their primary sequence, in which seven regions of 20–24 amino acid residues with aliphatic side chains are identifiable:
- These seven regions are proposed to be arranged in the phospholipid of the cell membrane with a highly recognisable pattern (Figure 2.2).

Table 2.1 Superfamilies of receptors

Receptor type	7-transmembrane receptors (7TMR)	Transmitter-gated channels (TGC)	Catalytic receptors	Nuclear receptors
Subunits	1/2	3/4/5	2/4	2
Structural domains	7 TM	2/3/4 TM	1 TM	0 TM DBD
Ligands	Small molecules, peptides, proteins	Small molecules	Peptides and proteins	Hydrophobic small molecules
Functional domain interactions	G-proteins	Ion channel	Docking proteins	Co-activators and RNA polymerase
Subunit size (aa)	318–1212	379–627	455–1382	410–777
Distribution	Ubiquitous	Nerve and muscle	Ubiquitous	Ubiquitous
Response times	10–60 s	< 1 s	10–6000 s	6000 s +

TM, transmembrane-spanning domain; DBD, DNA-binding domain; aa, amino acid length of peptide backbone.

Figure 2.2 A schematic representation of a human β_2-adrenoceptor. Identified in the figure are seven transmembrane domains in the plane of the plasma membrane phospholipid (defined by the two horizontal lines), defining three extracellular loops and an extracellular amino terminus as well as three intracellular loops and a cytoplasmic carboxy terminus. Also indicated is a disulphide bridge linking two extracellular cysteine residues and acylation of an intracellular cysteine residue, generating a fourth intracellular loop.

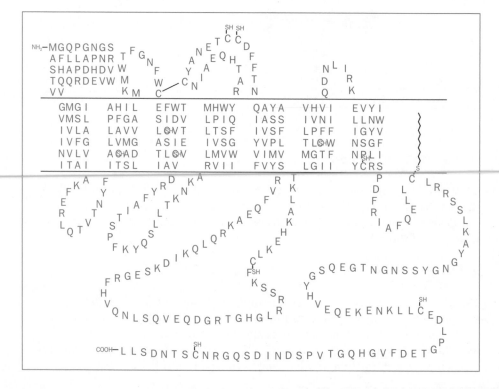

- This superfamily represents a significant portion of the human genome, estimated to be 1–2% of potential transcribed proteins.
- About half of these transcripts are gustatory or olfactory receptors and are unlikely to be useful drug targets.
- The remainder of the 7TMR (c. 350) represents the most readily 'druggable' proteins and they are targets for 25–60% of current drugs in clinical use.
- 7TMR may be classified on the basis of sequence similarities into three major classes:
  1. Class A, the rhodopsin-like family (300–450 amino acids), are numerically the largest group and include the receptors for the biogenic amines, such as the adrenoceptors and 5-hydroxytryptamine (5HT) receptors.
  2. Class B, the secretin receptor-like family, are larger in size (450–500 amino acids), respond mainly to peptide hormones and are primarily G_s-coupled (see Chapter 3).
  3. Class C, the metabotropic glutamate receptor family, are numerically the smallest family, although largest in size (950–1200 amino acids). They respond primarily to amino acids and divalent cations.

7TMR primarily (although not exclusively) evoke cellular responses via guanosine triphosphate (GTP)-binding proteins (G-proteins, see Chapter 3), hence the alternative nomenclature of G-protein-coupled receptors, or GPCR. Occupancy of the receptor by a suitable agonist leads to activation and dissociation of the G-protein from the receptor, in turn leading to the appropriate cellular cascade (Figure 2.3).

Figure 2.3 Agonist activation of a G-protein-coupled receptor. Binding of an agonist to an extracellular domain of the receptor causes a conformational change, which leads to dissociation of the alpha and beta:gamma subunits of the G-protein from the intracellular face of the receptor, each of which may mediate the cellular response to the agonist.

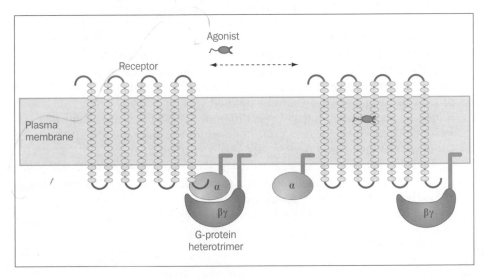

Sequence: structural elements of 7TMR

Figure 2.2 shows an arrangement of the amino acid sequence of a human β_2-adrenoceptor represented in two dimensions as a 'snake plot' to identify the suggested organisation of the receptor in the plasma membrane.

- Transmembrane domains comprise seven groups of 20–24 aliphatic amino acids (alanine, isoleucine, leucine and valine). These allow the receptor to be inserted in the hydrophobic environment of the phospholipid bilayer.
- At either end of the receptor are an extracellular amino terminal and an intracellular carboxy terminal, with three extracellular and three intracellular loops.
- For class A 7TMR, the binding site for ligands is within the plane of the plasma membrane, and so amino acid residues in this portion of the receptor have a major influence on ligand binding. For classes B and C 7TMR, binding of their natural ligands appears to be to the extended amino terminal.
- Attachment of a carbohydrate residue to an asparagine residue generates a glycoprotein (apparently a universal attribute for 7TMR) as the receptor is being synthesised in the rough endoplasmic reticulum. The precise function of glycosylation is unknown, but it might influence protein turnover and/or ligand binding.
- Attachment of an acyl group (usually palmitate or myristoate) often occurs at a cysteine residue of the carboxy terminal, to allow formation of a fourth, short intracellular loop, as the acyl group is sufficiently hydrophobic to allow insertion into the intracellular face of the plasma membrane.
- An influential posttranslational modification for every 7TMR in which the phenomenon has been investigated to date is phosphorylation, which occurs primarily at serine and threonine residues, but also at tyrosine residues.
- The impact of 7TMR phosphorylation is almost always to inhibit receptor function, by interfering with G-protein signalling, as a sequela of receptor desensitisation.
- Many, but not all, 7TMR also have disulphide bridges linking two extracellular cysteine residues to maintain a particular three-dimensional structure of the receptor.
- In recent years, it has become widely recognised that 7TMR function as oligomers; on occasion this is a phenomenon regulated by agonist binding. Frequently, this phenomenon is referred to as dimerisation, although the precise stoichiometry has yet to be defined.
- Heterodimers (combinations of two different 7TMR) have been identified:
  - $GABA_{B1}/GABA_{B2}$ form an obligate heterodimer, in that the $GABA_{B1}$ binds the ligand and $GABA_{B2}$ signals to the G-protein.
  - Opioid peptide receptors appear to be able to interact as KOP/MOP (κ/μ) and MOP/DOP (μ/δ) heterodimers, for which the resultant pharmacology is distinct from either partner alone.

'Unusual' 7TMR
Proteinase-activated receptors
- Ligands are enzymes (thrombin, trypsin, tryptase).
- Action involves hydrolysis of an *N*-terminal peptide unmasking a 'tethered ligand' to act within the plane of the plasma membrane.

Adiponectin receptors
- These receptors are inverted in the plasma membrane, with an extracellular COOH terminus and intracellular NH_2 terminus.
- Coupling appears to be to adenosine monophosphate (AMP)-activated protein kinase, without the involvement of G-proteins.

ANPc receptors
- 'Catalytic/clearance' receptor – 1TM
- Evidence for activation of $G_{i/o}$-proteins.

Calcitonin receptors and receptor activity-modified receptors (RAMPs)
- The calcitonin receptor is encoded by the gene *CALCR*, which is a classical 474 amino acid 7TMR. The endogenous peptide agonists have the potency order calcitonin > amylin. The receptor couples to both G_s- and $G_{q/11}$-proteins.
- Co-expressed with a 122 aa, single transmembrane domain protein, receptor activity-modifying protein, RAMP1 changes the agonist potency order to amylin > calcitonin. The receptor only appears to couple through G_s-protein.

Transmitter-gated ion channels

Transmitter-gated channels (TGC) are expressed predominantly in excitable tissues and are associated primarily with neurotransmission. These ion channels are often clustered together at synapses to increase the efficiency of signalling by summation of responses. They are the most rapidly acting of the receptors, responding to the presence of agonist by opening an intrinsic ion channel with a timescale measured in milliseconds (Figure 2.4). Transmitter-gated channels are multimeric with three, four or five subunits combining to form the active receptor.

The $GABA_A$ receptor is a useful example as it exhibits features common to many TGC.

$GABA_A$ receptors
Each individual subunit (of which 19 subtypes have been identified in mammals) is made up of four transmembrane domains, with both NH_2- and COOH-termini being extracellular (Figure 2.5). The large NH_2-terminus contains the binding site for the ligand, while the second intracellular loop is likely to be a site for interaction with docking proteins, which may regulate ion channel activity as well as positioning the receptor in a particular part of the plasma membrane.

Figure 2.4 Agonist activation of transmitter-gated channels. Binding of an agonist to an extracellular domain of the receptor causes a conformational change, which leads to opening of the ion channel and the consequent flow of ions across the plasma membrane. The precise spectrum of ions gated is determined by the amino acid residues lining the pore of the ion channel, while the direction of flow is determined by the gradient across the plasma membrane.

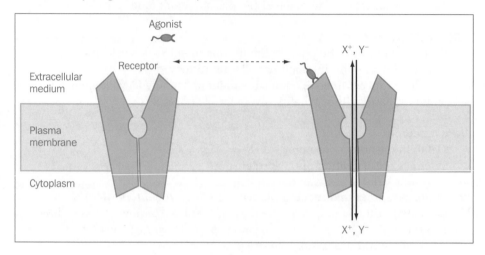

- GABA$_A$ receptors are probably the most abundant inhibitory receptor in the central nervous system (CNS).
- They respond to the inhibitory transmitter γ-aminobutyric acid (GABA) by gating chloride ions, leading to cellular hyperpolarisation and a reduction in transmitter release in neuronal cells.
- They are made up of five subunits (pentameric) arranged in a rosette or radially symmetrical fashion (Figure 2.6). The predominant GABA$_A$ receptor in the CNS is made of α_1, β_2 and γ_2 subunits, although with 19 subunits reported in mammals, the number of potential permutations and combinations is enormous. Binding of GABA appears to require α and β subunits, while benzodiazepine binding (see below) requires both α and γ subunits.
- Each subunit is made up of a glycosylated polypeptide that crosses the plasma membrane four times. As with the 7TMR, transmembrane regions 1, 3 and 4 are made up of high proportions of aliphatic amino acids, allowing insertion into the hydrophobic phospholipid environment of the plasma membrane. TM2, however, has a higher density of amino acids with positively charged side chains, which, when the channel is open, allows the rapid gating of anions across the plasma membrane.
- GABA$_A$ receptors are targets for barbiturates and benzodiazepines, which act at allosteric (other shape) regulatory sites distinct from the natural binding ligand on particular subunits of the GABA$_A$ receptor to enhance channel opening, thereby increasing the likelihood of depressing neurotransmission, leading to the hypnotic and antianxiety effects of these agents.

Figure 2.5 A schematic representation of an alpha subunit of a human GABA$_A$ receptor. Identified in the figure are four transmembrane domains in the plane of the plasma membrane phospholipid (defined by the two horizontal lines), defining an extracellular loop and extracellular amino and carboxy termini, as well as two intracellular loops. The agonist binding site is in the large extracellular amino terminus, while the second transmembrane domain lines the pore.

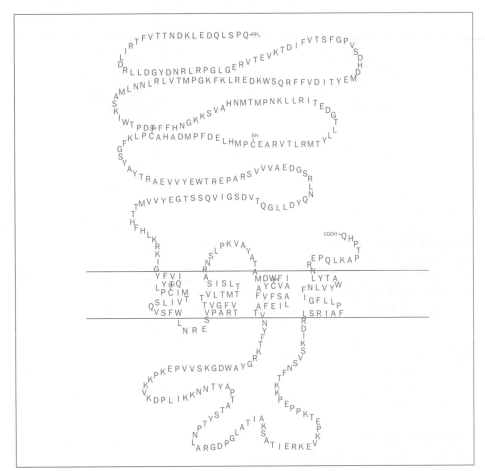

- In addition, particular neurosteroids, such as pregnenolone, act at GABA$_A$ receptors to enhance receptor function. The synthetic steroid alphaxolone targets these receptors to function as a veterinary anaesthetic.
- Penicillin, at high doses, can cause convulsions through blockade of GABA$_A$ receptors.
- Muscimol is found in *Amanita* mushrooms. It acts as a selective GABA$_A$ receptor agonist, causing hallucinations. Intriguingly, the same mushrooms produce a related chemical, ibotenate, which acts as an excitotoxic agonist at glutamate receptors (see below).

Figure 2.6 Agonist activation of *cys*-loop transmitter-gated channels. This bird's-eye view of the receptor depicts the rotational symmetry of the pentameric structure of *cys*-loop TGCs, as well as identifying that the second transmembrane domain (TM2) lines the pore of the channel. Agonist occupancy of (usually) two of the five subunits causes a conformational change in the receptor, particularly TM1 and TM3, thereby allowing TM2 to move apart from one another, opening the channel.

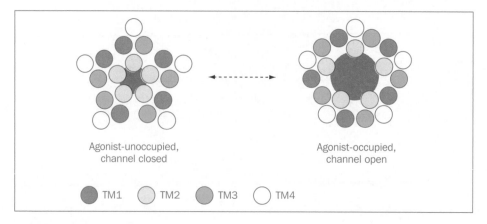

Other anion-gating TGC
Glycine receptors
- Glycine is a major inhibitory transmitter, particularly in the spinal cord, where receptor activation leads to Cl^- ion influx and neuronal hyperpolarisation.
- The antagonist strychnine acts at these receptors to cause convulsions (and possibly death through asphyxia or exhaustion).

5HT$_3$ receptors
- 5HT$_3$ receptors gate monovalent cations to cause neuronal hyperpolarisation and are the targets of many antiemetic antagonist drugs (e.g. ondansetron).

Cation-gating TGC
Glutamate (ionotropic) receptors
- Glutamate is the major excitatory neurotransmitter of the CNS with evidence for involvement at over 40% of synapses.
- Ionotropic glutamate receptors are divided into three main families on the basis of synthetic agents which discriminate them into *N*-methyl-D-aspartate (NMDA), kainate and α-amino-3-hydroxy-5-methylisoxazole-4-propionic acid (AMPA) receptors.
- Physiologically, AMPA receptors have prominent roles in excitatory transmission throughout the brain, and NMDA receptors in the hippocampus have a major role in the acquisition of learning and memory.
- Pathologically, NMDA receptors are associated with excitotoxicity (neuronal death due to excessive activation of excitatory receptors), leading to drug development of antagonists with, for example, therapeutic potential in ischaemic stroke or epilepsy. However, as yet, only a single, relatively weak NMDA receptor antagonist, memantine, has a clinical role in reducing

(slightly) the progressive neurodegeneration associated with Alzheimer's disease.

- Kainate receptors are also associated with excitotoxicity and they are the target for the shellfish-derived neurotoxin, domoic acid.

Acetylcholine (nicotinic) receptors

- Although by no means exclusive to skeletal muscle, nicotinic acetylcholine (nACh) receptors are the mediators of neurotransmission at the mammalian neuromuscular junction.
- They are also expressed at all autonomic ganglia and throughout the brain.
- At the neuromuscular junction, nACh receptors, when activated by acetylcholine, open to allow a rapid influx of sodium ions into the cell, leading to depolarisation and subsequent calcium influx and skeletal muscle contraction.
- In the CNS, nicotine inhaled from smoking cigarettes activates these receptors, particularly in the nucleus accumbens, to elicit reward but also dependency.

ATP (P2X) receptors

- Although adenosine triphosphate (ATP) is found at mM concentrations in every cell, with a primary role as an energy source, it also has roles as an excitatory neurotransmitter in the CNS.
- In the periphery, ATP is a co-transmitter with noradrenaline and acetylcholine in the sympathetic and parasympathetic nervous systems, respectively (see Chapter 6) and is an important component of non-adrenergic, non-cholinergic (NANC) neurotransmission.
- Given that one subtype of P2X receptor (the $P2X_7$ receptor) fails to show significant desensitisation and only responds to very high extracellular ATP concentrations, a role for P2X receptors in the necrosis associated with tissue damage has been suggested.
- Although P2X receptors have yet to be exploited in the clinic, a number of antagonists are in development, for the indications of chronic pain and bladder dysfunction, for example.

Catalytic receptors

Catalytic receptors are typically dimeric, cell surface proteins, with a single transmembrane domain separating an extracellular ligand binding site and an intracellular enzymatic activity (Figure 2.7). Receptors with extrinsic tyrosine kinase activity (including GFR and ErbB families for glial-derived neurotrophic factor and epidermal growth factor, respectively) and intrinsic protein serine/threonine kinase (phosphorylating) activity (including receptors for transforming growth factor-β) form minor subfamilies in this group.

Among the catalytic receptors, it is instructive to compare the two major signalling pathways of the particulate guanylyl cyclase (the enzyme that is responsible for cyclic guanosine monophosphate (cGMP) formation) and intrinsic protein tyrosine kinase activities associated with the ANP_A receptor (Figure 2.8) and the insulin receptor, respectively.

Figure 2.7 Agonist activation of catalytic receptors. Binding of agonist to the extracellular domain of the catalytic receptor causes a conformational change in the receptor leading to increased activity of the intracellular catalytic domain.

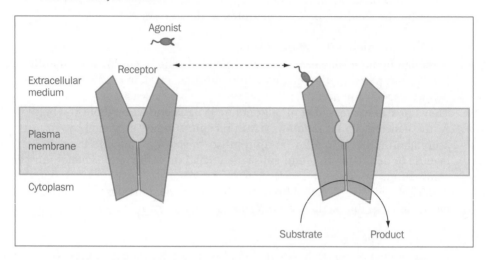

Atrial natriuretic peptide receptors

Atrial natriuretic peptide (ANP) receptors are a relatively small group of receptors; although recognised for some decades, their physiological and therapeutic roles have only recently been identified.

Features of the ANP receptor as an example of particulate guanylyl cyclases include:

- extracellular peptide-binding domain
- ligands include natriuretic peptides, guanylin and uroguanylin (short peptides, 28–50 amino acids)
- 1 TM-spanning region
- intracellular guanylyl cyclase activity leading to cyclic GMP (an intracellular messenger) formation
- dimerisation is obligatory for functional activity
- ANP secretion is stimulated by atrial wall stretch, possibly as a response to hypervolaemia
- elevated circulating ANP leads to:
  - vasodilatation by relaxing vascular smooth muscle through elevating intracellular cyclic GMP
  - increased urinary Na^+/K^+ excretion and diuresis through elevating intracellular cyclic GMP in the kidney
  - overall, a reduction in blood pressure is elicited.

Recombinant brain-type natriuretic peptide (BNP, nesiritide) has been approved for the treatment of acute decompensated congestive heart failure.

Insulin receptors

Amongst the tyrosine kinase receptors, the insulin receptor is unusual in that it is a heterotetramer linked covalently by disulphide bridges (Figure 2.9).

Figure 2.8 Particulate guanylyl cyclase activity. Binding of the peptide hormone atrial natriuretic peptide (ANP) to the extracellular binding domain of the ANP receptor enhances dimerisation of the receptor and stimulates enzymatic activity of the intracellular catalytic domain, increasing the conversion of guanosine triphosphate (GTP) to cyclic guanosine monophosphate (cGMP). Tissue responses (including vasodilatation and diuresis) to ANP receptor activation are mediated through raised intracellular cyclic GMP, and terminated through the action of phosphodiesterases, particularly phosphodiesterase (PDE5).

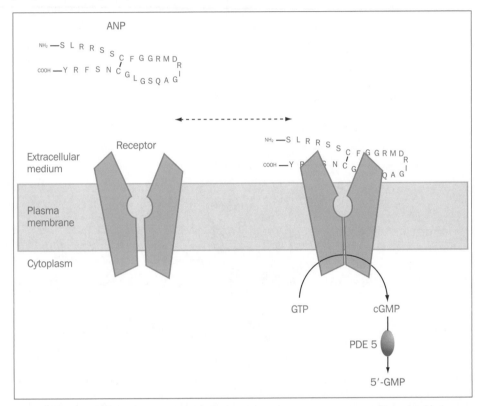

Features of the insulin receptor as an example of tyrosine kinase receptors include:

- extracellular protein-binding domain
- ligands are large peptides or proteins
- 1 TM spanning region
- intracellular protein tyrosine kinase activity
- oligomerisation as a requirement for functional activity.

Ligand binding at tyrosine kinase receptors leads to a cascade of events:

1. autophosphorylation of receptor
2. interaction with intracellular docking proteins
3. activation of effector enzymes:
   mitogen-activated protein (MAP) kinase cascade
   phospholipase C-γ (PLC-γ)
   phosphatidylinositol (PI) 3-kinase.

Figure 2.9 Schematic of the molecular mechanisms of insulin action. Insulin binding to the extracellular domain of the heterotetrameric insulin receptor causes a change in the intracellular enzymatic activity and autophosphorylation of the receptor. Accessory proteins are recruited through either phosphorylation or protein–protein interactions, leading to the cellular response. One major route of intracellular signalling involves activation of a phosphatidylinositol 3-kinase, generating phosphatidylinositol 3,4,5-trisphosphate (PIP$_3$), which in turn leads to activation of a variety of downstream enzymes, including protein kinase B (also known as Akt) and the zeta isoform of protein kinase C. PKC, protein kinase C; PDK, phosphoinositide-dependent kinase; PKB, protein kinase B.

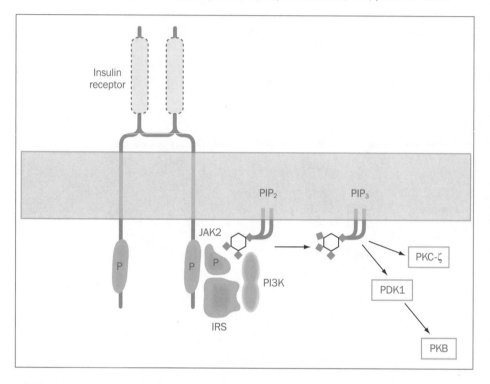

For the three major pathways of tyrosine kinase receptor signalling, the initial steps are identical, but subsequent pathways may differ between cell types and predominate at different periods following receptor activation, such that the overall cellular/tissue response is a composite of signalling through all three cascades.

There are several common features that are exhibited by docking proteins involved in the intracellular cascades regulated by tyrosine kinase receptors:

- Src homology domain 2 (SH2) recognises phosphotyrosine proteins generated by the activity of the receptor or of subsequent downstream tyrosine kinase activities.
- Src homology domain 3 (SH3) recognises proline-rich regions (e.g. PPPVPPRR) revealed upon conformational change in the target proteins.
- Signalling to the MAP kinase pathway, which can ultimately lead to changes in gene expression in the nucleus, involves a series of docking proteins which may alter the activity of a low-molecular-weight G-protein, Ras (see Chapter 3).

- In contrast, activation of the PLC-γ pathway is more direct, with few, if any, docking proteins involved in the recruitment and activation of PLC-γ from the cytosol to the plasma membrane.
- A major route for insulin receptor signalling relies on the activity of a kinase, which regulates phospholipid phosphorylation, PI 3-kinase (Figure 2.9).
- Following insulin binding to the extracellular face of the insulin receptor, tyrosine kinase activity on the intracellular face of the receptor leads to phosphorylation of the receptor itself, as well as insulin receptor substrate (IRS) and Janus-associated kinase 2 (JAK2).
- Together, these recruit to the plasma membrane and activate PI 3-kinase, which converts the substrate phospholipid, phosphatidylinositol 4,5-bisphosphate (PIP_2), to phosphatidylinositol 3,4,5-trisphosphate (PIP_3).
- This relatively rare phospholipid is able to activate an isoform of protein kinase C (zeta), and a phosphoinositide-dependent kinase, PDK1, which in turn activates protein kinase B (PKB).

In humans, insulin is secreted when circulating glucose levels are high and it acts to normalise blood glucose. At the cellular level, it is able to do this through the actions of PKB, which phosphorylates:
- GLUT4 glucose transporters, leading to increased glucose uptake from the blood into skeletal muscle and adipose tissue
- glycogen synthase kinase, leading to increased glucose storage through glycogenogenesis in skeletal muscle and liver
- phosphofructokinase, leading to increased glucose utilisation through glycolysis.

Nuclear receptors

Sequence homology studies indicate the presence of 48 nuclear receptors in the human genome, of which 24 have identified endogenous ligands. The remaining 24 are referred to as orphan receptors, with no suggested endogenous agonists. It has been surmised that these orphans are purely transcription factors without receptor function and that the nuclear receptors with defined endogenous ligands have simply evolved from analogous proteins, having developed the capacity for agonist recognition.

Two major families can be distinguished: class I and class II.

Class I: steroid hormone nuclear receptors
- Receptors for oestrogen (ERα and ERβ), progesterone (PR), androgen (AR), mineralocorticoids (MR) and glucocorticoids (GR).
- Ligand-dependent, in that gene transcription cannot proceed in the absence of agonist.
- In the absence of agonist, these receptors are bound to chaperone proteins in the cytoplasm.
- Homodimerisation is required for the receptor function to be evoked.

Class II: non-steroid hormone nuclear receptors

- Include receptors for thyroid hormone (TRα and TRβ), peroxisome. proliferator-activated (PPAR), vitamin D (VDR) and retinoic acid (RAR)
- Ligand-independent activation of gene transcription appears to take place.
- In the absence of agonist, these receptors are bound to co-repressor proteins in the nucleus.
- Homo- and heterodimerisation may take place, allowing receptor function to be evoked.

Steroids are dealt with in more detail in Chapter 33.

Nuclear receptor signalling involves:

- diffusion of hydrophobic agonist across cell membrane
- displacement of chaperone/co-repressor
- formation of receptor dimers
- interaction with DNA and other transcription factors
- zinc fingers, specialised parts of the DNA-binding domain (DBD) in activated receptor interact with genome (Figure 2.10).

Figure 2.10 A schematic of the portion of human peroxisome proliferator-activated receptor α (PPARα) generating the zinc fingers. Formed during the synthesis of the PPARα protein in the endoplasmic reticulum, the zinc atom co-ordinates with four cysteine residues to generate a three-dimensional structural motif for DNA-binding proteins. These are thought to allow insertion into the DNA double helix, allowing recruitment of additional proteins to regulate gene transcription.

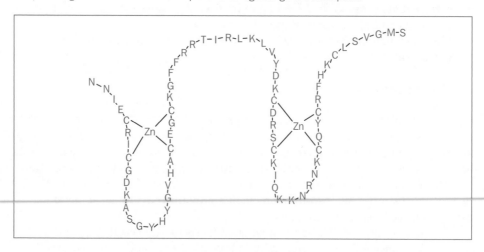

- The nuclear receptor binds to response elements (DNA consensus sequences) in the promoter region of target genes upstream of the coding region. Multiple response elements increase the recruitment of activated nuclear receptors and the likelihood of transcription of the target gene.
- Most response elements have an element of duplication to allow binding of the dimeric activated receptor:
  - oestrogen response element (ERE): AGGTCAnnnTGACCT or AGAACAnnnTGTTCT (i.e. an inverted palindrome, that is, the reverse strand of DNA shows the complementary sequence that is an inverse)

- peroxisome proliferator response element (PPRE): AGGTCAnAGGTCA or TGACCTnTGACCT (i.e. a repeat).
- They require co-activators for gene transcription.
- Nuclear receptors bound to hormone response elements recruit other proteins which modulate gene transcription.
- Amongst these, chromatin remodelling is a key event.
- Histone acetylation promotes DNA separation from histones and augments gene transcription.
- Co-activator proteins permit/enhance gene transcription:
  - histone acetyltransferases (HAT)
- Co-repressor proteins prevent/reduce gene transcription:
  - histone deacetylases (HDAC).

PPARs
- Peroxisomes – locus of fatty acid β-oxidation.
- Peroxisome proliferator-activated receptors – PPARs.
- Three subtypes: α, β (δ) and γ.
- Upon activation, form heterodimers with retinoid X receptors (RXR).
- Act at genome as transcription factors.

Bezafibrate, ciprofibrate, fenofibrate, gemfibrozil
- Used in treatment of hyperlipidaemias.
- PPARα agonists.
- Cause upregulation of lipid-metabolising enzymes, leading to decreased low-density lipoprotein (LDL: 'bad') cholesterol and increased high-density lipoprotein (HDL: 'good') cholesterol.

Rosiglitazone, pioglitazone
- Thiazolidinediones used in treatment of type 2 diabetes mellitus.
- PPARγ agonists.
- 'Master' regulator of adipocyte differentiation.
- Recovery of insulin sensitivity.
- PPRE, the peroxisome proliferator response element, regulates transcription of:
  - liprotein lipase, leading to an increased hydrolysis of triglycerides
  - hydroxyglutarylmethyl-coenzyme A (HMG CoA) synthetase, leading to an increased ketogenesis
  - cytochrome P450IVA6, leading to increased fatty acid ω-oxidation in microsomes
  - acyl-CoA oxidase, leading to increased fatty acid β-oxidation in peroxisomes.

A number of therapeutic/pharmacological targets commonly referred to as receptors are devoid of signalling and are therefore more correctly described as binding sites. For example,
- LDL receptors: LDLs transport cholesterol around the blood for incorporation in cell membranes and as a precursor of steroids (see Chapter 33).

- Elevated levels of LDLs are a risk factor for atherosclerosis.
- In the case of the LDL receptor, apolipoprotein B100 on the surface of the receptor is the primary point of attachment, although apolipoprotein E also shows some binding capacity.
- The LDL receptor is a member of a family of lipoprotein-binding single transmembrane domain glycoproteins expressed on the cell surface in the region of coated pits.
- Once LDL is bound to the LDL receptor, a number of adaptor proteins allow endocytosis (internalisation) to the lysosome to free up the cholesterol and to hydrolyse the proteins for recycling.

- Fibrinogen receptors: glycoprotein IIb (GPIIb) and GPIIIa (integrins) are components of the platelet surface which bind coagulation factors, including fibrinogen, as well as von Willebrand factor and fibronectin.
  - There is evidence for signalling enacted by integrins, although the precise manner of protein tyrosine kinase activation remains unclear, so the assignment of receptor function remains premature.
  - Fibrinogen, a hexameric protein secreted by the liver as a precursor of a clotting factor (see Chapter 15), allows bridging of platelets to occur, through multivalent interaction with GPIIb/IIIa.
  - Exposure and activation of GPIIb/IIIa is a late step in platelet activation and relies on phospholipase A_2-mediated activation.
  - GPIIb/IIIa can be blocked by eptifibatide, which has efficacy in the treatment of unstable angina and for reducing clotting and ischaemic episodes during coronary balloon angioplasty.

KeyPoint

- Receptors, especially the 7TM superfamily are the most widely clinically exploited drug targets.

Potential essay topic

Compare and contrast the signalling pathways associated with the four superfamilies of receptors.

chapter 3
G-proteins and their downstream signalling cascades

G-proteins are guanine nucleotide-binding proteins which are involved in signal transduction. They may be divided into heterotrimeric (made up of 3 subunits) G-proteins, which relay signals from cell surface 7-transmembrane receptors (7TMR: see Chapter 2), and low-molecular-weight or small, monomeric G-proteins, which are more associated with the action of catalytic receptors.

Heterotrimeric G-proteins

Structure
Heterotrimeric G-proteins are associated with the intracellular face of the plasma membrane. Their role is to provide and regulate the connection between 7TMR and their effector enzymes.
- Three separate subunits, α, β and γ, make up the G-protein, with 15 α (35–45 kDa), 5 β (21 kDa) and 13 γ (15 kDa) subunits identified in the human genome.
- Heterotrimeric G-proteins are most commonly named on the basis of the α subunit (e.g. G_s rather than $Gα_sβγ$) and divided into four families, dependent on structural similarities and the subsequent signalling pathway activated (Table 3.1).
- β and γ subunits are effectively a single inseparable entity once synthesised.
- For a long time, Gβγ subunits were considered to be relatively homogeneous, but recent evidence suggests a relatively modest variability in function.
- The α and γ subunits are anchored in the plasma membrane by the attachment of a hydrocarbon chain (see below).

The G-protein cycle
There are alternative models of the G-protein cycle. For instance, some 7TMR appear to 'pre-couple' to G-proteins, while others require agonist occupancy in order for this to occur.
- In the generalised version of the model presented here (Figure 3.1), the resting state of the receptor is unbound to either agonist or G-protein, which is an intact heterotrimer, where the α subunit has guanosine diphosphate (GDP) bound.

Table 3.1 Families of heterotrimeric G-proteins

G-protein	Effector enzyme	Second-messenger	Example agonists	Receptor
Gαs	Adenylyl cyclase stimulation	cAMP	Adrenaline 5HT Histamine	β-adrenoceptor 5HT$_4$ H$_2$
Gαi	Adenylyl cyclase inhibition, K$^+$ channels, Ca^{2+} channels	cAMP (inhibition), βγ subunits	Acetylcholine Histamine Noradrenaline 5HT	Muscarinic (M$_2$) H$_3$ α$_2$-adrenoceptor 5HT$_1$
Gαq	Phospholipase C	IP$_3$, DAG, Ca^{2+}	Acetylcholine Noradrenaline 5HT Histamine	Muscarinic (M$_1$ and M$_3$) α$_1$-adrenoceptor 5HT$_2$ H$_1$
Gα12	Rho GEF	Rho	Thrombin	Thrombin receptor

cAMP, cyclic adenosine monophosphate; 5HT, 5-hydroxytryptamine; IP$_3$, inositol 1,4,5-trisphosphate; DAG, diacylglycerol.

Figure 3.1 A schematic representation of the G-protein cycle. In this theoretical model, agonist binding to the 7-transmembrane receptor (7TMR) generates a transient high-affinity state of the receptor, allowing guanosine triphosphate (GTP) to exchange for guanosine diphosphate (GDP) at the α subunit of the G-protein (top arrow). GTP binding causes the G-protein to dissociate into Gα and Gβγ subunits, both of which may dissociate from the receptor to mediate the cellular effects of the agonist (right arrow). The inherent GTPase activity of the alpha subunit generates a GDP-bound form of the G-protein (bottom arrow), allowing reconstitution of the receptor–G-protein complex (left arrow).

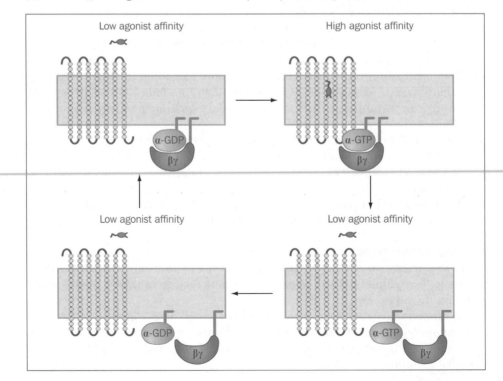

- Agonist binding to the receptor induces a conformational change which relays to the G-protein heterotrimer, stimulating exchange of GDP for guanosine triphosphate (GTP).
- This G-protein-bound complex of the receptor is transient and exhibits high affinity for the agonist.
- Rapidly thereafter, the receptor–G-protein complex dissociates and the G-protein itself dissociates into α-GTP and βγ subunits.
- These two components are independently capable of regulating intracellular second messenger cascades or cell surface ion channel activity.
- An inherent GTPase activity in the α subunit means that the GTP is hydrolysed to GDP, which allows reformation of the Gαβγ complex.

G-protein families

- G-proteins fall into four families, defined by the α subunits Gαs, Gαi, Gαq and Gα12 (Table 3.1).
- In general:
  - G_s-coupled receptors enhance cardiac muscle contractility, relax smooth muscle and enhance neurotransmitter release.
  - $G_{i/o}$-coupled receptors inhibit cardiac contractility, contract smooth muscle and inhibit neurotransmitter release.
  - $G_{q/11}$-coupled receptors contract smooth muscle and enhance neurotransmitter release.
  - $G_{12/13}$-coupled receptors stimulate chemotaxis and shape change.

Regulation of adenylyl cyclase activity and cAMP levels by G_s and G_i

- Nine isoforms of membrane-associated adenylyl cyclase have been identified, with a common structure; two repeats of six transmembrane domains, with each repeat apparently having an independent enzymatic activity for the conversion of adenosine triphosphate (ATP) to cyclic adenosine 3′,5′-monophosphate (cAMP) when stimulated by α_s-GTP (Figure 3.2).
- α_i-GTP, in contrast, evokes an inhibition of adenylyl cyclase activity.
- Elevated cAMP levels activate protein kinase A (PKA, cAMP-dependent protein kinase), thereby leading to the phosphorylation of numerous target proteins.
- PKA is unusual amongst protein kinases, in that activation leads to dissociation of regulatory and catalytic subunits from the functional heterotetramer (the majority of protein kinases contain regulatory and catalytic domains in a single protein).
- Phosphodiesterases catalyse the hydrolysis of cAMP to form 5′-AMP, which is inactive as a stimulus of PKA.
- In addition to phosphodiesterase (PDE) activities, the effects of cAMP can also be terminated by export out of the cell.
- Multidrug resistance proteins (MRP) 4, 5, 8 (also known as ABCC4, 5, 11) are responsible for efflux of cAMP:

Figure 3.2 Cyclic adenosine monophosphate (cAMP) turnover. Binding of agonist to a Gs-coupled receptor generates a guanosine triphosphate (GTP)-bound form of the α subunit (αs-GTP), which activates membrane-bound adenylyl cyclase activity. This catalyses the conversion of adenosine triphosphate (ATP) to cAMP, which activates protein kinase A (cAMP-dependent protein kinase), leading to dissociation of regulatory subunits (bound to cAMP) and catalytic subunits, which migrate through the cytoplasm to phosphorylate and regulate numerous proteins, leading to the cellular effect.

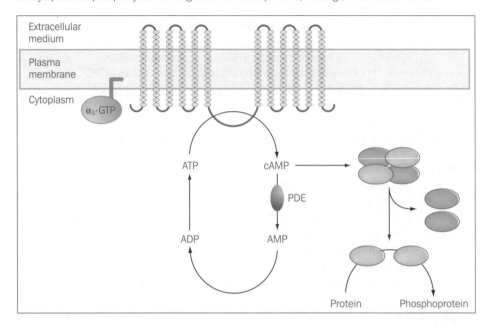

- The MRPs are members of the ATP-binding cassette (ABC) family that also includes CFTR (ABCC7) and P-glycoprotein (ABCB1) (see Chapter 4).
- The precise significance of this efflux is unclear.

Regulation of adenylyl cyclase activity

- $G\alpha_s$ stimulates all isoforms.
- $G\alpha_i$ inhibits AC 1, 3, 5, 6 (although not all isoforms have been tested).
- The plant-derived terpene forskolin stimulates all isoforms (except AC 9).
- Adenosine and deoxy derivatives acting at the intracellular P-site inhibit all isoforms, but only at elevated levels; this is proposed to be a means of conserving ATP levels in pathophysiological situations such as hypoxia/ischaemia where intracellular adenosine levels rise hugely.
- Different isoforms of adenylyl cyclase can be regulated by other signalling molecules, allowing a mechanism for convergence of signalling between cAMP-stimulating receptors and other signalling systems (a very common phenomenon known as signal transduction cross-talk).
  - Calcium ions enhance activity of AC 1, 3, 8 and inhibit activity of AC 5, 6, 9.
  - Gβγ subunits enhance activity of AC 2, 4 and inhibit activity of AC 1.
  - Protein kinase C (PKC)-dependent phosphorylation enhances activity of AC 1, 2, 3, 5, 7 and inhibits activity of AC 4, 6.

- cAMP-dependent protein kinase-mediated phosphorylation inhibits activity of AC 5, 6 and thereby represents a negative-feedback mechanism for limitation of cAMP production.

cAMP hydrolysis and its regulation

- cAMP-specific PDE activities: PDE2, PDE3, PDE4, PDE7, PDE8.
- Non-specific PDE activities (also hydrolyse cyclic guanosine monophosphate (cGMP)): PDE1, PDE10, PDE11.
- Phosphodiesterases, like adenylyl cyclase activities, are also convergence points for signal transduction cross-talk:
  - Intracellular calcium ions elevated by Gq-coupled receptors or by calcium-gating receptors increase PDE1 activity, thereby decreasing cAMP (and cGMP) levels.
  - cGMP increases generated by nitric oxide or particulate guanylyl cyclase activation stimulate PDE2 activity (thereby decreasing cAMP levels) or inhibit PDE3 activity (thereby increasing cAMP levels).
  - ERK1/2 (extracellular signal-regulated kinase 1/2, also known as p42/44 mitogen-activated protein kinase)-mediated phosphorylation, evoked by catalytic receptor activation, increases PDE4 activity, thereby decreasing cAMP levels.
  - Phosphatidic acid, evolved from phospholipase D activation, increases PDE4 activity, thereby decreasing cAMP levels.
- cAMP-dependent protein kinase-mediated phosphorylation increases PDE4 activity, thereby decreasing cAMP levels and acting as a negative-feedback mechanism for limitation of the duration of cAMP action.

Gs-protein signalling in the sympathetic nervous system

In the sympathetic nervous system (see Chapter 6), release of adrenaline leads to activation of β-adrenoceptors and the consequent elevation of intracellular cAMP. Thus, circulating adrenaline leads to:

- increased cardiac muscle contractility (β_1–AR) through phosphorylation and activation of cardiac calcium channels
- vasodilatation of skeletal muscle vascular smooth muscle (β_2–AR) through phosphorylation and inhibition of myosin light-chain kinase (MLCK)
- dilatation of bronchial smooth muscle (β_2–AR) through phosphorylation and inhibition of MLCK and phosphorylation and inhibition of calcium channels
- mobilisation of lipid in adipocytes (β_3–AR) through phosphorylation and activation of hormone-sensitive lipase
- mobilisation of glucose in the liver (β_2–AR) through phosphorylation of phosphorylase and glycogen synthase, leading to activation and inhibition, respectively:
- Genomic effects of PKA:
  - migration of the catalytic subunit to nucleus
  - phosphorylation and activation of cyclic AMP response element binding (CREB) protein
  - binding of phospho-CREB to CREs on many genes

- initiation/inhibition of gene transcription can be a mechanism of desensitisation (e.g. suppression of β-adrenoceptor and initiation of PDE4 gene transcription is a molecular mechanism of adaptation following protracted stimulation of β-adrenoceptors).

Gβγ: adenylyl cyclase-independent effects of G_i

- Aside from inhibiting adenylyl cyclase activity, G_i also has other functions.
- Evidence from the use of pertussis toxin (see below) indicates that G_i is a major source of Gβγ subunits, presumably due to its abundance and high rate of turnover compared to other G-proteins.
- Accordingly, agonist occupancy of G_i-coupled receptors can lead to the activation of a number of enzymes and ion channels, even (at first sight, paradoxically) adenylyl cyclase and phospholipase C (PLC).
- In nervous tissues, a major influence of G_i-coupled receptors is the inhibition of transmitter release, which is mediated by a stimulation of potassium ion efflux (leading to hyperpolarisation; Figure 3.3) and/or an inhibition of voltage-activated calcium channels.

Figure 3.3 K$^+$ channel action. In many excitable cells, such as neurones, smooth and cardiac muscle cells, the predominant mechanism of Gi signalling is through opening of cell surface potassium channels. Both guanosine triphosphate (GTP)-bound αi and Gβγ subunits are able to activate the potassium channel, leading to cellular hyperpolarisation.

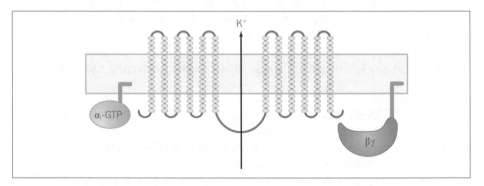

- This route of signalling is the molecular mechanism of action of numerous 7TMR, including α$_2$-adrenoceptors, GABA$_B$, A$_1$ adenosine, 5HT$_1$, mu, delta and kappa opioid peptide and CB$_1$ cannabinoid receptors.
- In cardiac tissue, both α$_i$-GTP and Gβγ appear to open potassium channels (Figure 3.4), the molecular mechanism of action of M$_2$ muscarinic acetylcholine and A$_1$ adenosine receptor activation.
- It has been suggested that the Gβγ regulation of potassium channels in the heart at rest is the mechanism of action of M$_2$ and A$_1$ receptors, while the α$_i$-GTP inhibition of adenylyl cyclase is the mechanism of action of these receptors upon sympathetic stimulation, when β-adrenoceptors are activated (i.e. antiadrenergic action).

Figure 3.4 Gαi action. In many cells, the predominant mechanism of action of Gi-coupled receptors is to inhibit adenylyl cyclase activity through the guanosine triphosphate (GTP)-bound form of the alpha subunit of Gi. ATP, adenosine triphosphate.

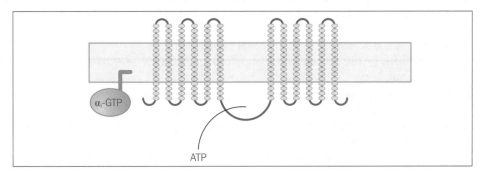

β-adrenoceptor kinase (βARK)

- Of major functional significance for Gβγ subunit signalling is the activation of G-protein-coupled receptor kinases (GRKs), in particular, GRK2 or β-adrenoceptor kinase (βARK).
- Initially identified as an element of the signalling cascade of β-adrenoceptors, it is likely that βARK activity is enhanced following agonist occupancy of many 7TMR.
- As the name suggests, once activated, βARK phosphorylates β-adrenoceptors.
- Of significance here is the profile of βARK action, in that the 'best' substrate appears to be the agonist-occupied β_2-adrenoceptor, where multiple serine/threonine residues in the extended cytoplasmic tail can be phosphorylated (see Chapter 2), presumably requiring an agonist-induced change in conformation for access to these amino acids.
- This phosphorylation can be very rapid (10–20 s) and occurs at high agonist concentrations, suggesting a synaptic relevance for the phenomenon (i.e. in close proximity to the higher concentrations of extracellular noradrenaline found in the body).
- As a result, a secondary protein, β-arrestin, binds to the intracellular face of the β_2-adrenoceptor, preventing coupling to the G-protein and promoting its internalisation by assisting the migration of the receptor to clathrin-coated pits.
- Once internalised, the receptor can be dephosphorylated and recycled back to the plasma membrane following acidification of the vesicle (endosome, presumably inducing a conformational change in the receptor) and the action of a phosphoprotein phosphatase (PP2B, calcineurin).
- The internalised receptor has also been suggested to couple to an enhancement of mitogen-activated protein kinase activity (particularly, ERK1/2).
- Overall, therefore, this route of signalling allows rapid termination of excessive signalling through the β-adrenoceptor, and may even change the downstream signalling cascade.

G_i-protein signalling in the parasympathetic nervous system

In the parasympathetic nervous system, acetylcholine release from nerve terminals acts on muscarinic acetylcholine receptors.

- In the heart, this leads to decreased cardiac muscle contractility, by two mechanisms:
  - increased K^+ efflux reduces basal contractility
  - reduced cAMP has antiadrenergic effects and reduces excessive contractility.
- On adjacent sympathetic nerve terminals, this leads to decreased transmitter release:
  - increased K^+ efflux results in membrane hyperpolarisation and reduced transmitter release.
- This mode of action is mimicked by a wide array of other G_i-coupled receptors:
  - noradrenaline/α_2AR; histamine/H_3; 5HT/5HT$_1$; dopamine/D_2; opioids/ MOP, KOP, DOP; GABA/GABA$_B$; cannabinoids/CB$_1$; adenosine/A_1; glutamate/mGlu$_2$.

G_t and the regulation of retinal cGMP levels

Although the majority of responses evoked by 7TMR through the activation of G-proteins are slower than those evoked by transmitter-gated channels (see Chapter 4), vision is an exception, with responses being registered on a millisecond timescale (Figure 3.5).

Figure 3.5 Transducin function. In the retina, light converts 11-*cis*-retinal to all-*trans*-retinal, leading to activation of the 7-transmembrane receptor rhodopsin. This activates the G-protein transducin, Gt, leading to activation of a heterotetrameric phosphodiesterase (PDE5). This reduces cellular levels of cyclic guanosine monophosphate (cGMP), leading to the closure of cyclic nucleotide-gated ion channels, in turn leading to hyperpolarisation of the cell.

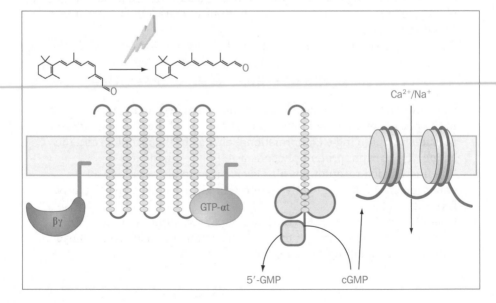

- Light enters the eye.
- Light causes conversion of 11-*cis*-retinal to all-*trans*-retinal (femtosecond timescale).
- It activates rhodopsin to switch on transducin (G_t).
- Transducin converts light-induced retinal switching to changes in ion fluxes by activating a cGMP phosphodiesterase (PDE6) in the plasma membrane, leading to a rapid reduction in intracellular cGMP levels, thereby switching off a cyclic nucleotide-gated (CNG) cation channel.
- Cones respond to bright light while rods respond to dim lighting.
- Cones express G_{t2}, while rods have G_{t1}.

Regulation of phospholipase C activity and calcium levels by G_q

- At least 13 isoforms of PLC have been identified, and these may be grouped into six families.
- The PLC-β family are associated with the cell membrane and are the targets of signalling from G_q-coupled 7TMR.
- PLC-γ isoforms are initially cytosolic and brought to the cell membrane following activation of particular catalytic receptors.
- PLC-δ isoforms are thought to be recruited to the cell membrane as a means of prolonging or sustaining the signalling via G_q-coupled 7TMR.
- Small G-proteins Ras and Rho (see below) are thought to be cellular activators of PLC-ε, while the most recently identified families ζ and η are incompletely characterised.
- Upon activation, PLC hydrolyses the minor membrane phospholipid (~0.1% of total membrane phospholipid) phosphatidylinositol 4,5-bisphosphate (PIP_2) to produce two second messengers, 1,2-diacylglycerol (DAG) and inositol 1,4,5-trisphosphate (IP_3).
- DAG is hydrophobic and remains in the membrane, whereas IP_3 is water-soluble and is able to migrate into the cytoplasm (Figure 3.6).
- DAG activates PKC, thereby leading to the phosphorylation of numerous target proteins, while IP_3 allows the release of calcium from intracellular stores by acting on intracellular IP_3 receptor ligand-gated channels.
- Elevation of intracellular calcium ions has regulatory effects on a wide range of cellular proteins (see below).
- Both IP_3 and DAG can be modified for recycling to PIP_2 or converted to other active entities.
- Extrusion of IP_3 out of the cell also occurs, but the mechanism and physiological relevance are obscure.

PIP_2 action and metabolism

PIP_2 is synthesised from phosphatidylinositol 4-phosphate (PIP) through the action of a selective kinase, PIP 5-kinase (PIP5K).

- Phosphatidic acid, small G-proteins ARF and Rho enhance PIP5K activity and increase PIP_2 levels.
- PKA-dependent phosphorylation inhibits PIP5K activity to prevent reformation of PIP_2.

Figure 3.6 Phosphatidylinositol (PI) turnover. Binding of agonist to a Gq-coupled receptor generates a guanosine triphosphate (GTP)-bound form of the α subunit (αq-GTP), which activates membrane-bound phospholipase C activity. This catalyses the conversion of phosphatidylinositol 4,5-bisphosphate (PIP$_2$) to diacylglycerol, which activates protein kinase C, leading to the phosphorylation and regulation of numerous proteins, leading to the cellular effect. At the same time, inositol 1,4,5-trisphosphate (IP$_3$) formation causes calcium release from intracellular stores. Sequential dephosphorylation of IP$_3$ allows reformation of membrane phosphatidylinositol, which is acted upon by specific kinases to form PIP$_2$. ER, oestrogen receptor.

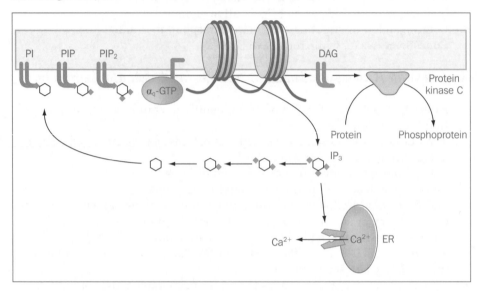

PIP$_2$ functions as an anchoring point or regulatory influence in the membrane for a number of cellular proteins:

- phospholipase D2, which migrates from the cytosol to the membrane upon uncovering of PIP$_2$
- the ion channel receptor TRPV1, which is tonically inhibited by PIP$_2$, allowing the channel to be sensitised by agonists at G$_q$-coupled receptors, such as bradykinin, histamine and PGE$_2$.

Aside from hydrolysis by PLC, PIP$_2$ is the substrate for an additional enzyme, phosphatidylinositol 3-kinase (PI3K):

- PI3K activity produces phosphatidylinositol 3,4,5-trisphosphate (PIP$_3$).
- PIP$_3$ is a poor substrate for PLC.
- PI3K activity is enhanced by tyrosine kinase catalytic receptors (see Chapter 2).
- PIP$_3$ can be dephosphorylated by phosphatase and tensin homologue (PTEN), an enzyme which undergoes a loss-of-function mutation in a very high proportion of human cancers at advanced stages (see Chapter 32).

Regulation of phospholipase C

- Similarly to adenylyl cyclase, different isoforms of PLC can be regulated by other signalling molecules, allowing a mechanism for convergence of signalling between Gq-coupled receptors and other signalling modalities:

- $G\alpha_q$ family increases activity of all isoforms of PLC-β.
- Calcium ions are required for catalytic activity of PLC-β, γ and δ isoforms, and are probably the major physiological form of regulation of PLC-δ activity.
- $G\beta\gamma$ subunits increase PLC-β1, β2, β3, δ1, η2 activity.
- Ras increases PLC-ϵ1 activity.
- cAMP increases PLC-ϵ1 activity through an unusual exchange factor, Epac.

Diacylglycerol metabolism

- DAG kinase:
  - forms phosphatidic acid
  - CTP transferase allows production of CDP-DAG, the precursor for reformation of phosphatidylinositol, which is sequentially phosphorylated by 4-kinase and 5-kinase enzymes to produce phosphatidylinositol 4,5-bisphosphate, the substrate for PLC
- DAG lipase:
  - forms 2-arachidonoylglycerol (2AG) , the 'best' candidate for an endogenous cannabinoid receptor agonist
  - thought to be a mechanism underlying the phenomenon of depolarisation-evoked suppression of excitation, whereby high concentrations of a stimulatory transmitter (e.g. glutamate or acetylcholine) enhance phosphoinositide turnover, leading to formation of 2AG in the postsynaptic specialisation. This (somehow) exits the cell and acts on CB_1 cannabinoid receptors on the presynaptic nerve ending to reduce transmitter release.

Inositol 1,4,5-trisphosphate metabolism

- IP_3 3-kinase:
  - forms inositol 1,3,4,5-tetrakisphosphate (IP_4), itself an agent which regulates calcium ion levels in the cytosol.
- IP_3 (and other inositol polyphosphate) phosphatases:
  - eventually form inositol phosphate, the substrate for inositol monophosphatase (IMPase)
  - IMPase is susceptible to uncompetitive blockade by Li^+ ions ($\sim$ 1 mM)
  - that is, Li^+ binds to (and inhibits) the enzyme–substrate complex, but not the enzyme alone
  - therefore, increased substrate concentrations lead to an increased degree of inhibition
  - effect is most profound with most active cells
  - the 'best' treatment for bipolar disorder (manic depression) is Li^+
  - dosing needs tight regulation (narrow therapeutic window)
  - desired plasma concentrations are 0.4–1 mM (12 hours after dose on days 4–7), with 2 mM considered overdosage.
- The current theory of lithium action in bipolar disorder:
  - Li^+ targets overactive neurones in cerebral cortex
  - Li^+ inhibits IMPase
  - Li^+ depletes inositol

- Li$^+$ prevents resynthesis of PIP$_2$
- Li$^+$ prevents formation of IP$_3$ and DAG
- overactive neuronal activity is decreased selectively, without affecting normal activity.

DAG action

- Targets of PKC action – a few examples:
  - smooth-muscle MLCK, phosphorylation of which on the appropriate residues leads to increased contractility
  - selected isoforms of phospholipase A$_2$, phosphorylation of which leads to increased arachidonic acid production, in a manner enhanced synergistically by elevated calcium ions and Gβγ
  - parietal cell proton pump (H$^+$/K$^+$-ATPase), phosphorylation of which leads to increased gastric acid secretion.

Calcium action

Elevation of intracellular calcium ion levels can influence the activity of very many enzymes and ion channels (see Chapter 4).

- Calcium-stimulated enzymes – a few examples:
  - protein kinases
    PKC (selected isoforms)
    calcium/calmodulin-activated protein kinase
    MLCK
  - phosphoprotein phosphatases
    PP2B or calcineurin
  - proteinases
    calcium-activated neutral proteases (calpains) are non-lysosomal intracellular cysteine proteases
  - phospholipases
    phospholipase A$_2$ (selected isoforms)
    PLC
  - endothelial and neuronal nitric oxide synthases
  - phosphodiesterases and adenylyl cyclases (see above).
- Almost all of these actions are mediated through calcium binding to a low-molecular-weight calcium-binding protein called calmodulin.

G$_{12/13}$–protein-coupled receptor signalling

- The signalling cascade involving activation of this class of G-protein, which is activated following agonist action at 7TMR for thrombin and lysophosphatidic acid, is the most recently identified of the routes of G-protein signalling and so it is likely that its broader significance has yet to be fully appreciated.
- It appears to have importance in cytoskelal rearrangements associated with responses such as cell migration (e.g. chemotaxis), morphological changes (e.g. platelet membrane ruffling) and smooth-muscle contraction.

- Intriguingly, there is evidence that $G\alpha_{12}$ and $G\alpha_{13}$ have distinct subcellular locations and perform distinct functions.
- Agonist occupancy of $G_{12/13}$-coupled receptors leads to activation of one of three RGS-type (see below) proteins, termed Rho guanine nucleotide exchange factor p115 (p115RhoGEF), leukaemia-associated RhoGEF (LARG) or PDZ domain-expressing RhoGEF (PDZRhoGEF) (Figure 3.7).
- This, in turn, activates the small G-protein Rho (see below).
- Rho-GTP switches on the activity of a number of enzymes directly and indirectly, principally Rho kinases (Rho-associated kinase 1 and 2, ROCK1 and 2), PLC-ε1, JNK (Janus-activated kinase, a member of the mitogen-activated protein kinases), phosphatidylinositol 4-phosphate 5-kinase, MYPT and phospholipase D (Figure 3.7).

Figure 3.7 Gα12 action. Binding of agonist to a G12-coupled receptor generates a guanosine triphosphate (GTP)-bound form of the α subunit (α12-GTP), which activates a guanine exchange factor for the low-molecular-weight G-protein, Rho. Activated Rho (RhoGTP) can activate multiple enzymes, either directly or indirectly, including phospholipase D (PLD), leading to the cellular effect. PIP5K, PIP 5-kinase; PLC, phospholipase C; JNK, Janus-activated kinase.

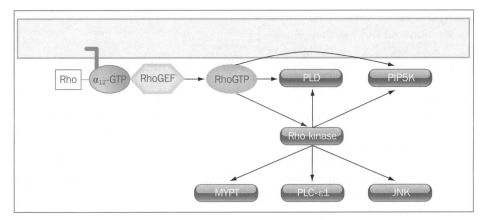

Small G-proteins

Low-molecular-weight or small G-proteins (20–25 kDa) can be divided into at least five groupings: Ras, Rho, Ran, Rab and Arf. Small G-proteins undergo a simpler version of the G-protein cycle compared to heterotrimeric G-proteins, whereby the resting state of the G-protein binds GDP. Activation causes exchange of GTP for GDP, leading to a cascade of intracellular signalling, terminated by inherent GTPase function of the G-protein.

- The Ras family couples catalytic receptors to the activation of mitogen-activated protein kinases (MAPK, particularly ERK1/2) and has, therefore, a putative role in regulating cellular proliferation. Mutations of Ras family members, particularly HRAS, are found in about one-third of human solid tumours.

- Rho (Ras homology, also known as ARH, Aplysia Ras-related homologue) is proposed to have a major role in regulating cell morphology through an influence on the cytoskeleton. Rho couples $G\alpha_{12/13}$ heterotrimeric G-proteins to Rho kinase activity. Rho kinases can, by phosphorylating and inhibiting the function of myosin light-chain phosphatase (MLCP) and/or its endogenous inhibitor (MYPT), lead to a sustained contraction of smooth muscle. The Rho/Rho kinase axis regulation of myosin phosphorylation can also influence cell shape and movement, particularly in leukocytes.
- Ran regulates protein translocation across the nuclear membrane, with a particular role during mitosis.
- Rab and Arf G-proteins regulate membrane trafficking within the cell, in particular vesicle migration from the endoplasmic reticulum to the Golgi apparatus and plasma membrane. The Rab family has been suggested to control membrane recycling from cell surface to intracellular locations and back again.

Posttranslational modifications of G-proteins

Prenylation
- Unsaturated hydrocarbon chain
- Farnesyl (C16) or geranylgeranyl (C21)
- For Ras, Rab and Rho, attached at C-terminus cys-AAX (where A is an aliphatic amino acid, such as valine, leucine or isoleucine), prior to cleavage of AAX
- Anchors $G\gamma$ and low-molecular-weight G-proteins in the plasma membrane
- Activity of small G-proteins is dependent on prenylation and is an indirect means of regulating activity:
  - inhibition of farnesyl/geranylgeranyl availability through inhibition of hydroxyglutarylmethyl-coenzyme A (HMG CoA) reductase by statins limits the function of small G-proteins
- Essentially irreversible.

Methylation
- For Ras, following prenylation and proteinase uncovering of a C-terminal cysteine, methylation allows capping
- Essentially irreversible.

Acylation
- Myristoate (tetradecanoate, C14)
  - G_i family ($G\alpha_{i/o/t}$) but not $G\alpha_s$
  - ARF small G-protein
  - attached at N-terminal gly
- Palmitoylation
  - Ras and Rho small G-proteins
  - Attached to a cysteine residue in close proximity to the C-terminal
- Anchors $G\alpha$ and small G-proteins in membrane
- Reversible

- allows cycling and targeting of small G-proteins to different membranes in the cell.

Phosphorylation
- Many Gα subunits are substrates for protein kinases in vitro
- Attached at serine/threonine/tyrosine residues
- The functional impact of phosphorylation in intact cells/tissues is unknown.

Bacterial toxins
- *Bordetella pertussis*
  - the causative agent of whooping cough
  - transmitted as an inhaled aerosol
  - causes aqueous hypersecretion in the lungs
- *Cholera vibrio*
  - the causative agent of choleric dysentery
  - transmitted by drinking contaminated water
  - causes aqueous hypersecretion in the bowel
- Both toxins have adenosine diphosphate (ADP)-ribosylation activity
  - use NAD + protein as co-substrates
- Pertussis toxin targets Gi
  - permanent off-switch
- Cholera toxin targets Gs
  - permanent on-switch
- Adenylyl cyclase activity is elevated by both agents in the epithelial cells of their respective organ targets
- Epithelial water secretion is increased.

Modulation of G-protein function: GAPs, GEFs and GDIs

- In addition to direct receptor regulation of the heterotrimeric G-proteins, the function of both these and the small G-proteins is acutely regulated by ancillary proteins which enhance (GEF) or inhibit (GAP, GDI) G-protein activity.
- For those small G-proteins which are frequently mutated in human tumours (particularly Ras), the mutations frequently occur in parts of the proteins influenced by GAPs, GEFS and GDIs, thereby interfering with the cell's potential influence over their activity.

GTPase-activating proteins (GAPs)
- GAPs enhance the enzymatic function of the small G-proteins and Gα subunits of the heterotrimeric G-proteins.
- Many of the GAPs which activate the latter group have additional functions in the cell, not least as effector enzymes for 7TMR signalling, including PLC-β and adenylyl cyclase.
- A series of over 20 related proteins, termed regulators of G-protein signalling or RGSs, have been identified, which target primarily $G\alpha_i$ and $G\alpha_q$ families.

- In enhancing the GTPase function of G-proteins, GAPs increase the turnover of the G-protein cycle and so are capable of terminating agonist effects at the level of the G-protein.
- Switch off G-protein signalling cascades by accelerating termination of Gα activity (thereby sequestering Gβγ).

GTP exchange factors (GEFs)

- GEFs are proteins which enhance the exchange of GTP for GDP upon activation of either class of G-protein.
- For heterotrimeric G-proteins, the 7TMR itself acts as a GEF.
- GEFs increase the likelihood of GTP:GDP exchange at Gα subunits.
- They amplify signalling through G-protein.
- Their primary role in the activation of small G-proteins:
  - They can be used as a route of coupling heterotrimeric G-proteins to activation of small G-proteins.
- Examples include:
  - RhoGEFs, such as p63RhoGEF, link G_q and Rho signalling
  - SOS (son of sevenless) links protein tyrosine kinase receptors to Ras.

Guanine nucleotide dissociation inhibitors (GDIs)

- GDIs are proteins which bind preferentially to the GDP-bound form of small GTPases, such as Rho and Rab, preventing guanine nucleotide exchange and also prevent association of the small G-protein with the plasma membrane.
- They are mainly associated with Rho and Rab families of small G-proteins.
- GDIs stabilise the GDP-bound, inactive form of the G-protein.
- They increase dissociation of the G-protein from the plasma membrane, possibly by interacting with prenylation tag.
- GDIs are proposed to be inhibited by proteins in the plasma membrane (integrins?) involved in cell–cell interactions or cell signalling cascades.

KeyPoint

- The four families of heterotrimeric G-proteins are mediators of cell signalling linking the 7TMR superfamily to intracellular signalling cascades.

chapter 4
Ion channels and transporters

- Ion channels allow regulated flow of ions across membranes, both inside cells and across the cell membrane.
  - Since the cellular and organelle ion constitution can have profound effects on cellular activity, ion channels represent an important drug target.
- Transporters carry solutes across membranes which would otherwise be impermeable to them.
  - The majority of transporters make use of established ionic gradients (source of potential energy) to allow co-transport of the solute of interest.
- Although ion channels are present in every cell, cell surface ion channels are most commonly associated with nerve cell function, since the rapidity of neurotransmission relies on the opening and closing of ion channels.
- The amino acids that line the central pores through which the ions flow determine the selectivity of the channel.
- For example, amino acids with positively charged side chains (arginine and lysine) will reduce the flux of cations, such as Na^+, K^+ or Ca^{2+}, but promote the flow of anions, such as Cl^- or HCO_3^-.
- In the main, ion channels can be differentiated structurally and on the basis of how they are regulated.

Ion channels regulated from inside the plasma membrane

Intracellular ATP-regulated channels
- Intracellular adenosine triphosphate (ATP) can regulate particular ion channels in two ways: either as an intracellular ligand (K_{ATP} channels) or as an energy source to influence ion movements against a gradient.
- K_{ATP} channels are sensitive to intracellular levels of ATP and adenosine diphosphate (ADP), such that ADP causes the channel to close, while ATP allows the channel to open. In the pancreatic β-cell, low plasma glucose levels mean that intracellular ATP levels drop, while ADP levels rise.
- This balance of nucleotides causes the K_{ATP} channel to open and the efflux of K^+ ions causes β-cell hyperpolarisation and a reduction in insulin secretion.
- In contrast, high plasma glucose levels achieved after a meal cause intracellular ATP levels to rise, thereby closing the K_{ATP} channel.

- This allows the cell to depolarise and insulin secretion to take place, allowing the extraction of glucose from the plasma to take place.
- K_{ATP} channels are targets for oral hypoglycaemic agents (sulphonylureas), used in the treatment of type 2 diabetes mellitus, which enhance insulin secretion, such as glibenclamide, through blocking pancreatic β-cell K_{ATP} channels selectively.
- Nicorandil activates K_{ATP} channels selectively; in vascular smooth muscle, this allows vasorelaxation and relieves the symptoms of angina (see Chapter 13).

ATPases

Plasma membrane ATPases ('ion pumps') allow extrusion of ions against a gradient.

- Na^+/K^+-ATPases allow repolarisation of the plasma membrane after an action potential and are targets of cardiac glycosides, such as digoxin.
- H^+/K^+-ATPases in the parietal cells of the stomach are regulated by phosphorylation evoked by H_2 histamine, M_1 muscarinic acetylcholine and gastrin (CCK_2) receptors.
  - Activation of any of these receptors causes an increased gastric acid secretion.
  - These proton pumps are the targets of antiulcer drugs, such as omeprazole.
- The cystic fibrosis transmembrane regulator (CFTR) is a member of the ATP-binding cassette (ABC) family of transporters (see below) and is the common site of mutation in cystic fibrosis.
  - It functions as an ATPase, driving the efflux of anions, principally Cl^- and HCO_3^-.
  - Secretion of these ions into the lumen of the lungs or pancreas generates an osmotic gradient, which enables the secretion of water.
  - In cystic fibrosis, the absence of this aqueous secretion means that the mucus in the lungs and pancreas is excessively thick, preventing adequate gas exchange in the lungs and enzyme secretion in the pancreas, leading to the respiratory problems and malnutrition, respectively, exhibited by sufferers.

Vanilloid (TRPV1) and related receptors

- Transient receptor potential (TRP) channels were first identified in the visual system of the fruitfly, *Drosophila*. More recently, they have been identified as important regulators of mammalian neuronal function, particularly sensory neurones, as well as being responsible for regulating ion fluxes intracellularly.
- TRP channels are unusual in that they respond not only to small molecules, but also to changes in temperature, with particular channels being activated at low (<17°C, TRPA1), intermediate (<22°C, TRPM8; >24°C, TRPV4) and high (>43°C, TRPV1; >53°C, TRPV2) temperatures.
- TRPV1 (vanilloid) receptors respond to the pungent component of chilli peppers, capsaicin, which gives chillies and curries their spiciness, while

TRPM8 and TRPA1 respond to menthol, a component of skin care products that gives the sensation of cooling.

- The channels are highly expressed in sensory nerves and probably represent the body's temperature detectors.
- The endogenous ligand that stimulates TRPV1 receptor opening and the consequent gating of calcium ions appears to be anandamide, a fatty acid derivative first identified as an endogenous agonist of cannabinoid receptors. The channel is also highly sensitive to protons and its activity is greatly enhanced at pH <5. Anandamide is generated inside the cell and appears to act on the intracellular side of the TRPV1 receptor. Although the mechanisms of anandamide generation are incompletely defined, a key stimulus appears to be calcium influx, implying that TRPV1 receptors are involved in the prolongation of painful stimuli in primary afferent neurones, rather than in their initiation.
- Antagonists at the TRPV1 receptor are being developed as potential analgesics.
- Other members of the TRP families appear to function as store-operated calcium channels, responding to depletion of calcium from intracellular stores, thereby allowing receptor responses to be sustained. An unusual family member (TRPM7) has both ion channel and enzymatic function, leading to the novel descriptor, chanzyme.

Voltage-sensitive channels

Voltage-sensitive channels exist in one of three states: closed, open or inactivated.

Voltage-sensitive sodium (Na$_v$) channels
- These are responsible for the initiation of the action potential.
- They are composed of one α subunit, which forms the functional pore, and one or two regulatory β subunits. α subunits have 24 identifiable TM domains, divided into four homologous domains of six, with TM4 being positively charged and acting as the voltage sensor.
- Na$_v$ channels may be activated by veratridine, aconitine and scorpion toxin.
- Na$_v$ channels may be inhibited by:
  - local anaesthetics, such as procaine and novocaine
  - antiepileptics, such as phenytoin and carbamazepine.
- Some subtypes appear to be the molecular targets of the toxin derived from the puffer fish, tetrodotoxin, served in fugu restaurants in Japan.
- Some subtypes, prominently expressed in sensory nerves, are targets of drug development for the treatment of chronic pain.

Voltage-sensitive calcium (Ca$_v$) channels
- Voltage-sensitive calcium channels are responsible for calcium influx in excitable tissues, such as nerve and muscle. In nerves, they are commonly concentrated in the presynaptic nerve terminal, where they allow

depolarisation-evoked transmitter release. In the heart and vascular smooth muscle, they are targets for the dihydropyridine calcium channel antagonists used in the treatment of hypertension.

■ Voltage-sensitive calcium channels are divided into multiple subtypes (T, N, L, P, Q, R), based on biophysical differences.

Voltage-sensitive K$^+$ (K$_v$) channels

■ Voltage-sensitive K$^+$ channels repolarise the cell following an action potential and thereby limit the duration and frequency of depolarisation events.

■ Loss-of-function mutations are associated with arrhythmias and these HERG (human ether-a-go-go-related gene, originally defined in *Drosophila*) channels in cardiac cells are inhibited by a variety of chemicals, leading to QT interval prolongation and, hence, substantial failures in drug discovery programmes.

Voltage-sensitive Cl$^-$ (ClC) channels

■ Members of the ClC family of chloride ion channels are incompletely characterised and the association with currents observed in cells and tissues is poorly defined.

Second messenger-operated ion channels

Cyclic nucleotide-regulated

■ Cyclic nucleotide-gated (CNG) channels are found in the eye and nose, with major roles in visual and olfactory transduction (see Chapter 3).

■ Hyperpolarisation-activated, cyclic nucleotide-gated (HCN) channels are associated with pacemaker currents in excitable tissues, particularly in the heart and nervous system.

Calcium-activated K$^+$ (BK and SK channels) and Cl$^-$ (CaCC) channels

■ These are activated following elevation of calcium influx (often resulting from depolarisation), causing hyperpolarisation of the membrane, thus acting as a negative-feedback cycle.

■ The scorpion venom-derived charybdotoxin and iberiotoxin, as well as the bee venom-derived apamin, block calcium-activated potassium channels, contributing to the paralysing or painful effects of these agents.

M-current (G-protein-regulated)

■ M-currents are a subset of inwardly rectifying potassium channels (K$_{ir}$ 3.x), which are activated by G-proteins (with evidence for activation by both Gαi and G$\beta\gamma$ subunits).

■ They underlie the vagal inhibition of cardiac activity, coupling M$_2$ muscarinic acetylcholine receptors to membrane hyperpolarisation.

Intracellular channels

Calcium channels
- Inositol 1,4,5-trisphosphate (IP_3) and ryanodine receptors are responsible for the release of calcium from intracellular organelles, particularly on the endoplasmic or sarcoplasmic reticulum.
- IP_3, generated following activation of particular cell surface receptors, such as M_1 muscarinic acetylcholine, H_1 histamine receptors or α_1-adrenoceptors, acts at IP_3 receptors to cause a rapid increase in intracellular calcium ion concentrations to create, for example, smooth-muscle contraction.
- The action of IP_3 is enhanced at moderate, but inhibited at higher, intracellular calcium ion concentrations, presumably acting as a feedback inhibition cycle.
- Intriguingly, these higher concentrations of calcium cause ryanodine receptors to open on adjacent intracellular organelles, leading to a propagation of the calcium signal and a wave of calcium within the cell.
- The endogenous ligand of the ryanodine receptor has yet to be identified, but may turn out to be the novel second messenger, cyclic ADP ribose.
- Calcium is once more accumulated into these stores through a thapsigargin-sensitive Ca^{2+}-ATPase, known as SERCA or the sarcoplasmic/endoplasmic reticulum calcium ATPase. It has been hypothesised that the parasitic SERCA is the molecular target of the antimalarial drug, artemesinin.

Proton channels
- The regulation of intracellular proton fluxes, which are mediated through two distinct classes of ATPases, is an important part of organelle function.
- For mitochondria, the electron transfer chain of the inner mitochondrial membrane allows an accumulation of protons in the intermembrane space, generating a large electrochemical gradient.
- The F_0F_1-ATPase, which is inhibited by the antibiotic oligomycin, utilises this gradient to generate ATP from ADP and inorganic phosphate.
- V-ATPases, in contrast, use ATP to generate a proton gradient.
- This is exploited in lysosomes and endosomes to enhance enzyme function in these organelles.
- The degradative/recycling role of lysosomes, in particular, is dependent on an acidic organellar pH of *circa* 4–5, being optimal for the various lipases, glycosidases, proteases, phosphatases and nucleases contained therein.
- The low pH may also be useful in reducing the activity of enzymes involved in the normal function of any engulfed pathogen trapped in the lysosomes.

Plasma membrane transporters

- In nervous tissue, plasma membrane transporters allow cellular accumulation of neurotransmitters and neuromodulators, providing an opportunity for recycling or reducing extracellular levels of neurotransmitters to terminate neurotransmission.

- More generally, amino acid and nucleoside transporters are ubiquitous and allow accumulation of the precursors of protein and nucleic acid synthesis, respectively.

Excitatory amino acid transporters
- Excitatory amino acids, L-aspartate and L-glutamate, are major excitatory neurotransmitters with the potential for excitotoxicity (neuronal damage due to excessive cation, mainly Ca^{2+}, influx) at high concentrations.
- Glial versus neuronal:
  - Glial accumulation of glutamate is of high density and avidity, making use of sodium (and sometimes proton) gradient. It allows conversion of the potentially excitotoxic glutamate to the less toxic glutamine, which can be exported for accumulation in neurones and regeneration of glutamate in excitatory neurones. Alternatively, glutamine can be accumulated by inhibitory neurones as a precursor for γ-aminobutyric acid (GABA).
  - Neuronal accumulation of glutamate is of lower avidity, allowing for recycling or metabolism.

Monoamine transporters
- DAT, NET and SERT transport dopamine, noradrenaline (norepinephrine) and 5HT (serotonin), respectively.
- Monoamine transporters exploit the sodium gradient to carry monoamines into the cell for recycling or metabolism.
- They have significant clinical relevance as therapeutic targets:
  - DAT and NET also transport amphetamine, methamphetamine and MPP^+ (inhibitor of mitochondrial function derived from the neurotoxin MPTP, which causes a Parkinson's disease-like state)
  - DAT is inhibited by mazindol.
  - NET is inhibited by nisoxetine.
  - SERT also transports MDMA (3,4-methylenedioxymethamfetamine: ecstasy).
  - SERT is inhibited by the selective serotonin reuptake inhibitors (SSRIs; see Chapter 20) paroxetine, sertraline and fluoxetine.
  - Cocaine is a non-selective inhibitor of all three monoamine transporters.

Choline transporters
- Exploit the sodium gradient to carry choline into the cell for resynthesis of acetylcholine or for metabolism
- Are inhibited by hemicholinium-3.

Inhibitory amino acid transporters
- Glycine and GABA transporters exploit sodium gradients to allow cellular accumulation of inhibitory amino acids for recycling or metabolism.
- They play a major role in the termination of inhibitory tone.

Nucleoside transporters
- There are two main types, equilibrative and concentrative:
  - Equilibrative transporters (SLC29) carry nucleosides in either direction across the cell membrane, dependent on the nucleoside concentration gradient.
  - Concentrative transporters (SLC28) carry nucleosides into the cell, exploiting the sodium gradient.
- They transport all five nucleosides: adenosine, guanosine, thymidine, uridine, cytidine.
- Both types are exploited by antiretrovirals and anticancer agents: AZT, gemcitabine, didanosine, cladribine.

Gap junctions (connexins)
- Six connexin molecules form a connexon hemichannel, which co-ordinates with a hemichannel on an adjacent channel to form a gap junction.
- Gap junctions allow the movement of small solutes across plasma membranes.
- They allow non-synaptic communication between neurones.
- Solutes gated include inorganic ions, second messengers (such as cyclic adenosine monophosphate (cAMP) and IP_3), as well as many intracellular ions less than 1000 Da.
- Mutations in the genes encoding connexins appear to underlie some inherited disorders in the ear, vascular system and peripheral nervous system.
- Carbenoxolone, derived from the liquorice plant, is a relatively selective inhibitor.

Aquaporins
- At least one family member is found in every cell.
- Aquaporins are responsible for water transport across cell membranes.
- Some family members also transport glycerol (aquaglyceroporins).
- They are found in intracellular membranes as well as on the cell surface.
- Functional aquaporins are unusual structures; they are tetrameric, with each subunit of six TM domains acting as a separate pore.

Fatty acids
- Six fatty acid transport proteins (FATP) allow accumulation of fatty acids into cells, particularly adipocytes, skeletal muscle, cardiomyocytes, liver, kidney and brain.
- They appear to concentrate in close proximity to CD36, which binds oxidised low-density lipoproteins on the cell surface, acting as a relay to intracellular enzymes or receptors, such as the peroxisome proliferator-activated receptors (PPARs).

ATP-binding cassette transporters

ABC transporters are probably the largest family of membrane transporters, able to regulate the flow of a huge array of both endogenous and exogenous substances, primarily out of the cell. Structurally, they have two domains of usually six transmembrane-spanning regions (unusually up to 11), with one or two intracellular nucleotide-binding domains (NBD). These bind and hydrolyse ATP, generating the energy to extrude or accumulate solutes. In bacteria, prokaryotic orthologues allow accumulation of solutes, including carbohydrates, peptides and vitamins, and have also been hypothesised to export some antibiotics, leading to resistance.

- Six families of mammalian ABC transporters are defined, with a standard nomenclature of ABCA to ABCG.
- The ABCA family includes transporters for cholesterol and lipid efflux.
- The ABCB family includes ABCB1 (also known as P-glycoprotein and multidrug resistance protein 1), which exports a wide range of cytotoxic drugs, leading to resistance during cancer chemotherapy. For this reason, the ABCB1 is probably the most closely studied example of ABC transporters. ABCB11 exports bile salts in the liver; loss-of-function mutations are associated with intrahepatic cholestasis.
- The ABCC family (initially decribed as multidrug resistance proteins, MRPs) include transporters for leukotrienes (ABCC1), prostaglandins (ABCC4, MRP4), nucleosides and cyclic nucleotides (ABCC4 and ABCC5), as well as CFTR (ABCC7). Members of this family also confer sulphonylurea-sensitive ATP binding to the K_{ATP} channel family.
- The ABCD family transport lipids across peroxisomal membranes.

Intracellular transporters

In all cells, transporters allow the movement of metabolites from the cytosol into organelles:
- pyruvate as a substrate for oxidative phosphorylation in mitochondria
- phospholipids and proteins for degradation in lysosomes
- fatty acids for oxidation in mitochondria and peroxisomes.

Distinct transporters allow metabolites to be exported from organelles into the cytosol:
- mRNA for protein translation out of the nucleus
- ATP for energy out of mitochondria.

In neurones, specialised vesicular transporters distinct from cell surface transporters allow the concentration of transmitters in synaptic vesicles:
- monoamine transporters
- acetylcholine transporters
- glutamate transporters (v-Glut).

Key Points

- Ion channels and transporters are major targets for current and future drugs.
- They are found in every cell, but have major roles in the regulation of neuronal activity.
- They regulate extracellular, intracellular and organellar environments.

Self-assessment

1. **Omeprazole inhibits:**
a. Na^+/K^+-ATPase
b. sarcoplasmic/endoplasmic reticulum Ca^{2+}-ATPase
c. H^+/K^+-ATPase
d. K_{ATP} channels
e. CFTR

2. **AZT is a substrate for:**
a. nucleoside transporters
b. sarcoplasmic/endoplasmic reticulum Ca^{2+}-ATPase
c. dopamine transporters
d. Na^+/K^+-ATPase
e. CFTR

3. **Which of the following ion channels or transporters are activated by ATP?**
a. nucleoside transporters
b. sarcoplasmic/endoplasmic reticulum Ca^{2+}-ATPase
c. dopamine transporters
d. Na^+/K^+-ATPase
e. CFTR

4. **Which of the following ion channels or transporters are activated by calcium ions?**
a. nucleoside transporters
b. sarcoplasmic/endoplasmic reticulum Ca^{2+}-ATPase
c. IP_3 receptors
d. ryanodine receptors
e. CFTR

chapter 5
Quantitative pharmacology

- A crucial tenet of pharmacology is to show concentration (or dose) dependence of a drug. In order to allow efficient comparison of agents, drug actions are quantified.
- Three important characteristics of a drug can be identified:
  1. What effect does it have?
  2. How much drug is needed to see an effect?
  3. How big an effect does it have?
- The effect a drug has depends on the molecular targets with which it interacts (see Chapter 1). Most drugs alter activity of receptors, enzymes, transporters and/or ion channels. Here, we will consider primarily the interaction of drugs with receptors, although the majority of these principles are also applicable to drugs which act at other targets.

Drugs which alter receptor activity

- These drugs can enhance (agonists) or inhibit (antagonists) receptor activity.
- Agonists are agents which mimic the effects of the natural ligand:
  - They bind to a receptor and evoke a cellular response.
  - Usually the natural ligand is unstable, so synthetic agonists prolong response by resisting metabolism/uptake.
- Antagonists are agents which bind to a receptor *without* producing a response. It is important to note that they are *not* the opposite of agonists.
  - Since they occupy the receptor, they prevent the agonist from evoking a response.
  - Antagonists are inert, and can only produce effects by preventing the effects of an agonist.

Agonist activation of receptors: potency and efficacy

- It is possible to define three quantitative properties of agonists as they interact with receptors:
  1. affinity: how well the agonist binds to the receptor
  2. potency: how much is needed to cause the receptor to generate a response
  3. efficacy: how big the response generated by the agonist is.

Generating quantitative data for agonist action at receptors
  1. Agonist binds to the receptor.
  2. A conformational change in the receptor is evoked.

3. A signalling cascade is initiated.
4. This leads to a cellular/tissue response.

- This response is plotted on a semilogarithmic scale to generate a log concentration–response curve, which should follow a sigmoidal or S-shaped plot (Figure 5.1). Increasing the concentration of agonist (above a threshold) evokes a rapid increase in response, until the maximal response attainable is obtained, and the curve saturates.

Figure 5.1 A sigmoidal plot of agonist-evoked response. Note the logarithmic scale on the x-axis.

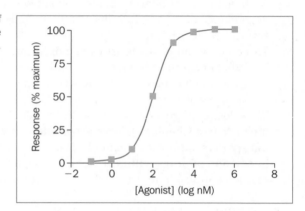

- The sigmoidal plot has four useful parameters (Figure 5.2):
  1. R_{min}, the response in the absence of agonist
  2. R_{max}, the maximal response to the agonist
  3. EC_{50}, the concentration of agonist which elicits half the maximal response to that agonist
  4. Hill slope, the steepness of the curve as it passes through the EC_{50} point.

Figure 5.2 The four-parameter logistic equation or sigmoidal plot.

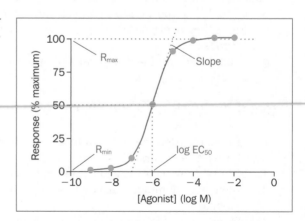

- The equation of the sigmoidal plot is based on the following:
  - y-axis is the response.
  - x-axis is the logarithm of agonist concentration
  - y starts at R_{min} and goes to R_{max} with a sigmoid shape:

$$Y = R_{min} + \frac{(R_{max} - R_{min})}{1 + 10^{((logEC_{50}-X).Slope)}}$$

- In practice, this equation is not consciously applied, but rather the parameters are derived from a graphical plot or with iterative curve fitting to a model using a computer program (e.g. GraphPad Prism).

Comparing agonist potencies

- Provided the same receptor is involved and an identical maximal response is obtained, agonist potencies can be compared quantitatively:

$$Relative\ potency = \frac{EC^1_{50}}{EC^2_{50}}$$

- These values are usually expressed as -fold:
  - Drug x is 30-fold less potent than drug y.
  - Drug y is 30-fold more potent than drug x.
- For example, Figure 5.3 illustrates a comparison between two agonists, which evoke an inhibition of spontaneous contractility in a cardiac muscle preparation.
- Agonist 1 causes a concentration-dependent inhibition of tone, starting from basal levels of 150 mg force to a maximal inhibition of 50 mg force. The maximal response evoked by agonist 1 is, therefore, -100 mg force. The potency of agonist 1, determined by the EC_{50} value, is 100 nM.
- Agonist 2 also causes a concentration-dependent inhibition of tone, starting from the same basal levels of 150 mg force, also reaching a maximal effect at 50 mg force. As with agonist 1, the maximal response evoked by agonist 2 is, therefore, -100 mg force. The potency of agonist 2, determined by the EC_{50} value, is 10 µM.
- The relative potency of the two agonists can be expressed in two ways:
  1. Agonist 1 is 100-fold more potent than agonist 2.
  2. Agonist 2 is 100-fold less potent than agonist 1.

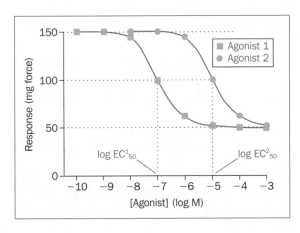

Figure 5.3 Relative potency of two agonists acting at the same receptor. In this plot, increasing concentrations of agonist 1 or agonist 2 evoke concentration-dependent inhibitions of cardiac muscle contractility.

- The same ratio can be applied to determine quantitatively the selectivity of an agent between two receptors.
  - For example, if drug NCE1 (novel chemical entity 1) has a potency at the H_1 histamine receptor of 50 nM and a potency at the M_1 muscarinic acetylcholine receptor of 1 µM, it can be said to be (1000/50) = 20-fold selective for H_1 histamine receptors.

Agonist efficacy

- Agonist efficacy is the ability of an agonist, once bound to the receptor, to evoke a response. It depends on two properties:
  1. the intrinsic efficacy of the agonist
  2. the tissue and response being studied. Given the phenomenon of signal amplification, where steps in a signal cascade allow sequential increases in the magnitude of a response, efficacy can appear to vary depending on the response being considered.

Reduced efficacy or partial agonists

- Some agonists occupy the receptor, but are unable to elicit the same maximal response seen with other agonists (Figure 5.4).

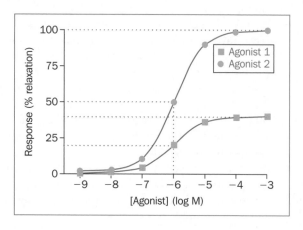

Figure 5.4 Partial agonism. Both agonist 1 and agonist 2 act through the same receptor to evoke relaxation of smooth muscle, and exhibit identical potency (log EC_{50} = −6). However, agonist 2 evokes a greater maximal response than agonist 1, indicating that agonist 1 is a partial agonist.

- These are described as partial agonists or, more correctly, agonists with reduced efficacy.
- Full agonists are able to occupy only a proportion of receptors to generate a maximal response:
  - The remaining unoccupied receptors are referred to as spare receptors and full agonists are described as having a receptor reserve.
  - Because a partial agonist has to occupy all the receptors in a tissue to generate a maximal response, partial agonists are described as having no receptor reserve.
- Although superficially a paradoxical statement, it is true to say that a partial agonist is not always a partial agonist, since the efficacy of an agonist can vary with the tissue studied or with the response investigated.

- Higher density of receptor expression or 'better' coupling of a receptor to the signalling cascade can enhance the apparent maximal response to a partial agonist.
- Signal amplification for more downstream parts of a signalling cascade means that maximal responses to partial agonists more closely approach those of full agonists.

Combining full and partial agonists

- A partial agonist can act functionally as both an agonist and an antagonist.
- In the absence of other agonists, it evokes a response, albeit not to the same maximal level as a full agonist.
- In the presence of a full agonist, it will inhibit the response to achieve a maximal response no different from the presence of partial agonist alone:
  - At a simple conceptual level, the partial agonist can occupy all the receptors without producing the optimal conformational change to elicit a maximal response.
  - In so doing, it can prevent the action of a full agonist, which would otherwise be able to produce a full response by occupying only some of the receptors.

Efficacy versus occupancy for a full agonist

- Agonist (abbreviated to A) binding to a receptor (abbreviated to R) is a dynamic equilibrium, where the agonist–receptor complex can be described by the term AR:

$$A + R \rightleftharpoons AR$$

- We can describe this equilibrium in exactly the same way that chemical equilibria are described, using an affinity constant, K_A, where:

$$K_A = \frac{[AR]}{[A].[R]}$$

- We can describe the fractional occupancy of the receptor (i.e. how much receptor is occupied by the agonist) using the term α in the same equation, with the free receptor concentration as $1 - \alpha$:

$$K_A = \frac{\alpha}{[A].(1 - \alpha)}$$

- This can be rearranged to allow determination of α, the fractional occupancy:

$$\alpha = \frac{[A].K_A}{1 + [A].K_A}$$

- From this equation, it is clear, therefore, that the degree of occupancy of a receptor is determined both by the affinity of the agonist for the receptor, K_A, and the concentration of the agonist, $[A]$.
- This equation has the form of a sigmoidal plot, when α, the fractional occupancy, is plotted against agonist log concentration, as can be seen in Figure 5.5 (circles).

Figure 5.5 Agonist occupancy and potency for a full agonist. The difference between concentrations of agonist needed to evoke half the maximal response and those needed to occupy 50% of receptors (in this case, 1000-fold) is an index of the efficacy of the agonist.

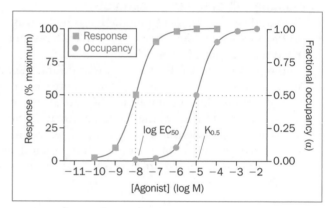

- From this graph, it is apparent that agonist occupancy of the receptor requires higher concentrations of agonist than are required to evoke a response (squares). As an illustration, it is informative to compare the half-maximal concentrations. Potency is determined as before, using the EC_{50} value, which in this example is 10 nM (log $EC_{50} = -8.0$). The concentration of agonist at half-maximal occupancy (where $\alpha = 0.5$), the $K_{0.5}$, is 10 µM (log $K_{0.5} = -5$). The difference between agonist occupancy and potency is an index of efficacy – in this case, 1000-fold.
- From the graph, it is also apparent that a sizeable response to the agonist can be achieved by occupying only a small proportion of the receptor. For example, consider the agonist concentration of 100 nM, at which a near-maximal response is elicited. At this concentration, only about 2% of the receptor is occupied by the agonist. The remainder of the receptor population (98% in this case) is referred to as spare receptors or the receptor reserve.

Efficacy versus occupancy for a partial agonist

- For a partial agonist, the occupancy curve will appear very similar to a full agonist; however, the potency curve is less left-shifted. Thus, the $K_{0.5}$ and EC_{50} values are much closer; efficacy is reduced (Figure 5.6).
- In this example, the occupancy of the receptor by the partial agonist has the same $K_{0.5}$ value as the previous full agonist (Figure 5.5); that is, 10 µM. However, the potency of the partial agonist is reduced compared to the full agonist, with an EC_{50} value of only 3 µM (log $EC_{50} = -5.5$).

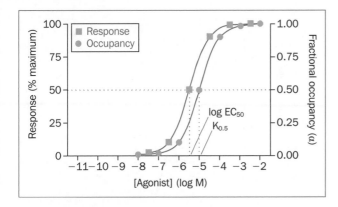

Figure 5.6 Agonist occupancy and potency for a partial agonist. The reduced ratio of EC_{50} and $K_{0.5}$ observed (threefold) compared to Figure 5.5 indicates the reduced efficacy of the partial agonist compared to the full agonist.

Partial agonists in the clinic

- It is sometimes useful to use a 'self-limiting' drug so that it achieves a measurable effect without producing the largest possible effect, which may be detrimental.
- Examples of partial agonists in the clinic include buprenorphine, which is used for the treatment of opiate addiction. The ability to elicit a modest stimulation of opioid receptors, while at the same time preventing the action of the more efficacious agonist morphine, is a useful outcome.

Antagonist occupancy of receptors: affinity estimation

- Antagonists are conventionally divided by pharmacologists into two types, where the nature of the antagonism is described to be either surmountable (competitive) or non-surmountable.
- An antagonist which occupies the binding site and prevents the agonist from binding and, hence, generating a response is described as a competitive or surmountable antagonist:
  - Increasing agonist concentration will overcome (surmount) the antagonist blockade.
- Non-surmountable antagonists can exert their effects through two routes.
  1. A competitive, irreversible antagonist binds initially at the same site as the agonist, but then covalently attaches to the receptor. In effect, therefore, a particular proportion of the receptors becomes permanently unavailable for interaction with the agonist, leading to a depression of the maximal response evoked by the agonist.
  2. An alternative mechanism of action of a non-surmountable antagonist would be to bind at sites other than the agonist binding site and prevent receptor function allosterically. This phenomenon is best characterised at transmitter-gated channels (see Chapter 4), where the cognate transmitter binds to one subunit of the functional receptor and other subunits express binding sites for modulatory agents.
- Increasing the agonist concentration fails to overcome the antagonist blockade completely (Figure 5.7), resulting in what pharmacologists usually refer to as non-competitive blockade.

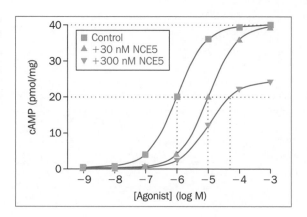

Figure 5.7 Non-competitive antagonism of agonist-evoked cyclic adenosine monophosphate (cAMP) accumulation.

- Antagonists which are only effective after agonist activation of the receptor are termed use-dependent antagonists or, by analogy with enzyme inhibitor interactions, uncompetitive antagonists.
- Conventional pharmacological analysis does not distinguish between use-dependent and non-competitive antagonists. This requires a kinetic approach, best typified by electrophysiological investigations, such as patch clamp analysis.
- To distinguish competitive and non-competitive antagonists, a range of concentrations of antagonist are employed to determine whether a linear increase in antagonist concentration evokes a linear increase in the concentrations of agonist needed to overcome the antagonist (Figure 5.8).

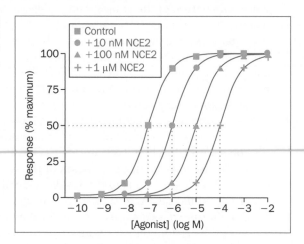

Figure 5.8 The use of increasing concentrations of antagonist to investigate the surmountable nature of the antagonist.

- In Figure 5.8, the EC_{50} value for agonist-evoked responses in the absence of antagonist is 100 nM (log EC_{50} = -7). In the presence of 10 nM NCE2, the EC_{50} value is increased to 1 µM (log EC_{50} = -6). Increasing the antagonist concentration 10-fold to 100 nM NCE2 results in a 10-fold increase in the concentration of agonist required to achieve the same response (EC_{50} value of 10 µM, log EC_{50} = -5). Increasing the antagonist concentration 100-fold to 1 μM NCE2 results in a 100-fold increase in the concentration of agonist required to achieve the same response (EC_{50} value of 100 μM, log EC_{50} = −4).

■ The graphical plot used to display these data is named after an early pharmacologist, Hans Schild. Because the range of concentrations of antagonists needed to generate appropriate increases in agonist potencies is usually conducted over three orders of magnitude, the axes of the Schild plot are generated as log values (Figure 5.9).

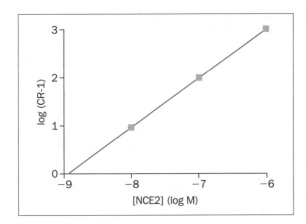

Figure 5.9 A Schild plot of novel chemical entity 2 (NCE2), a competitive antagonist, indicated by the slope of unity.

■ For a competitive antagonist, the slope of the line of best fit, which joins the points, should be unity.

■ The point where the line of best fit intercepts the x-axis (that is, where the concentration ratio is extrapolated to null) is a measure of the antagonist affinity for the receptor. Numerically, this is the log of the antagonist dissociation constant (K_i value). Usually, the negative value of the intercept is reported as a pA_2 value (typically in the range 4–12). In Figure 5.9, the pA_2 value is 9.95, equivalent to a K_i value of 1 nM.

■ Non-competitive antagonists will generate lines of best fit with slopes below unity. Under these conditions, it is not appropriate to compute pA_2 values.

The Gaddum transformation

■ In practice, to save time when multiple antagonists are being investigated, it is possible to make an assumption that all the agents are competitive.

■ The magnitude of the increase in agonist concentrations required to achieve the same level of response in the presence of a fixed concentration of antagonist is dependent on two factors:
  1. the affinity of the antagonist for the receptor
  2. the concentration of the antagonist.

■ Thus, for a known concentration of antagonist, determining the relative increase in agonist concentration will allow calculation of the antagonist affinity constant:
  ● For the same level of response, the same occupancy of the receptors is needed.

- Therefore, the degree of occupancy (usually referred to as α, the fractional occupancy) is the same at 50% maximal response.
- Previously, we defined fractional occupancy using the equation, where [A1] is the agonist concentration in the absence of antagonist:

$$\alpha = \frac{[A1].K_A}{1 + [A1].K_A}$$

- We can extend this to include a factor for the antagonist concentration, [B], which incorporates the antagonist affinity, K_B, agonist concentration in the presence of antagonist, [A2]:

$$\alpha = \frac{[A1].K_A}{1 + [A1].K_A} = \frac{[A2].K_A}{1 + [A2].K_A + [B].K_B}$$

- Although this looks complicated, it is simply relating the degree of occupancy, α, of the receptor by the agonist to four parameters: the agonist affinity and concentration (K_A and [A]) and the antagonist affinity and concentration (K_B and [B]).
- The equation can be rearranged and simplified:

$$\frac{[A2]}{[A1]} = [B].K_B + 1$$

- The left-hand side is usually abbreviated to CR, the concentration ratio, similar to the potency ratio we defined above, allowing us to calculate K_B, the antagonist affinity constant:

$$K_B = \frac{(CR - 1)}{[B]}$$

- Since an antagonist affinity constant is the inverse of an antagonist dissociation constant, K_i, which is measured in 'real' units of concentration, the more common version is:

$$K_i = \frac{[B]}{(CR - 1)}$$

- This can be rearranged to allow generation of an apparent pA_2 (or pK_i) value:

$$pK_i = \log(CR - 1) - \log[B]$$

where:
- CR is the concentration ratio of the EC_{50} value of agonist in the presence of antagonist divided by the EC_{50} value of agonist in the absence of antagonist.

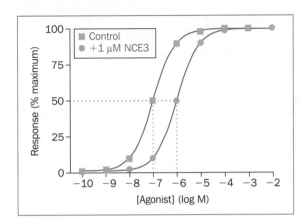

Figure 5.10 Antagonist novel chemical entity 3 (NCE3)-evoked shift in agonist concentration–response curve.

- [B] is the antagonist concentration.
- In the example illustrated in Figure 5.10, the EC_{50} value for the agonist-evoked response in the absence of other ligands is 100 nM (log EC_{50} = −7). In the presence of 1 μM NCE3, the agonist concentration–response curve appears shifted to the right 10-fold, with an EC_{50} value of 1 μM (log EC_{50} = −6). From this, a concentration ratio of 10 is rapidly calculated, allowing completion of the Gaddum transformation:

$$K_i = \frac{[B]}{(CR - 1)} = \frac{1 \times 10^{-6}}{(10 - 1)} = \frac{1 \times 10^{-6}}{9} = 1.1 \times 10^{-7} M$$

- Or, in its logarithmic form:

$$pK_i = \log(CR - 1) - \log[B] = \log(10 - 1) - \log 1 \times 10^{-6} = \log 9 - -6 = 6.95$$

The null method

- The Gaddum and Schild approaches to determining antagonist affinities work well with traditional pharmacological assays such as isolated tissue contractile response studies, where (commonly) four simultaneous preparations are run in parallel. One tissue can function as the control, where agonist cumulative concentration–response curves are constructed in the absence of antagonist. The other three tissues are exposed to three different antagonist concentrations and the same concentrations of agonist are used to construct three further concentration–response curves. The contractile response is monitored in real time and so results are rapidly visualised.
- Studies of receptor-evoked second-messenger generation are usually conducted in a very different manner with multiple (typically 24–48, but exceptionally 96 or more) tissue or cell samples exposed simultaneously. Assessment of the results is usually delayed because of the method of quantification of the second messenger, which often involves estimation of radioisotopes in a scintillation counter. In the null method of antagonist affinity estimation (after Leff–Dougall), an agonist concentration–response

curve is conducted with each sample being exposed to different concentrations of agonist, with multiple repeats (replicates of 2–4) at each concentration. At the same time, an antagonist concentration–response curve is constructed in the presence of a fixed concentration of agonist, C. The agonist concentration chosen is one which evokes a response between 60% and 85% of the maximal response (i.e. on the linear part of the curve). The IC_{50} value for antagonist inhibition of the agonist-evoked response is calculated by graphical means. The concentration of agonist, C', which evokes a response which is half that evoked by the fixed concentration of agonist, C, is also calculated. The K_i value can then be calculated using the following equation:

$$K_i = \frac{IC_{50}}{C/C' - 1}$$

- If the use of pK_i values is preferred, this equation may be rearranged as follows:

$$pK_i = \log(C/C' - 1) - \log IC_{50}$$

Figure 5.11 The null method for calculating antagonist dissociation constants. This method makes the assumption that the antagonist is competitive. cAMP, cyclic adenosine monophosphate.

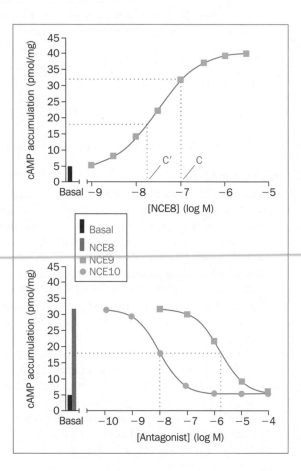

- In the example shown in Figure 5.11, basal levels of cyclic adenosine monophosphate (cAMP) are 5 pmol/mg protein, and are stimulated in the presence of NCE8 in a concentration-dependent manner, with an EC_{50} value of 30 nM (log $EC_{50} = -7.5$). The concentration of NCE8 chosen for subsequent examination of potential inhibitors is 100 nM, and is designated C. Since this concentration of NCE8 evokes an accumulation of cAMP of 32 pmol/mg protein, it is necessary to calculate the accumulation of cAMP equivalent to half that level of stimulation, taking into account basal levels:

$$\frac{32-5}{2} + 5 = \frac{27}{2} + 5 = 13.5 + 5 = 18.5$$

- Therefore, the concentration of NCE8 which evoked an accumulation of 18.5 pmol/mg was determined as 20 nM (equivalent to -7.7 log M).
- Using the fixed concentration of 100 nM NCE8, C, the antagonists NCE9 and NCE10 evoked concentration-dependent inhibitions of cAMP accumulation (Figure 5.11). The IC_{50} values derived from the graph were 10 nM for NCE10 (log $IC_{50} = -8$) and 1.8 µM for NCE9 (log $IC_{50} = -5.75$).
- The K_i value for NCE9 may be calculated as follows:

$$K_i = \frac{IC_{50}}{C/C' - 1} = \frac{1.8 \times 10^{-6}}{100/20 - 1} = \frac{1.8 \times 10^{-6}}{5 - 1} = \frac{1.8 \times 10^{-6}}{4} = 4.5 \times 10^{-7} M$$

- The pK_i value for NCE10 may be calculated as follows:

$$pK_i = \log(C/C' - 1) - \log IC_{50} = \log(100/20 - 1) - -8 = 8 + \log(5-1) = 8 + \log(4) = 8 + 0.6 = 8.6$$

Defining whether a novel chemical entity is an agonist or antagonist

- Add increasing concentrations of the NCE to the tissue and check for an effect (response).
- If it evokes a response, it is an agonist, so plot the concentration–response curve for the NCE.
- If the NCE has no effect, it might be an antagonist.
- Add a known agonist and repeat the concentration–response curve to the NCE.
- If it inhibits the effect to the agonist, it is an antagonist.
- Alternatively, add the NCE to the tissue and add the agonist in increasing concentrations.
- Plot a concentration–response curve to the agonist and determine whether the NCE has changed the agonist concentration–response curve.

Radioligand binding

Principle

- The principle of radioligand binding (or a more recent variant with a fluorescently tagged ligand) is relatively simple:
  - Label a ligand with a tag (an isotope, a fluorescent moiety or an enzyme).
  - Allow it to come into contact with (bind to) the receptor.
  - Separate bound ligand from free ligand (most often this separation is conducted by filtration).
  - Measure how much is bound.
- The ligand should ideally have some selectivity for the target, although it is sometimes advantageous (and potentially cheaper) to have a ligand which binds to all subtypes of a given receptor:
  - It should also show reasonable stability, both chemically and biochemically.
  - It should exhibit ease of handling and preparation. The most common isotopes in use for radioligand binding are β-emitters ($[^3H]$, $[^{14}C]$ and $[^{35}S]$) or the γ-emitter $[^{125}I]$.
- Radioligands bind to target receptor and other sites:
  - Examples include other receptors, enzymes, phospholipid, filter paper, and incubation vessel.
  - Two parallel conditions should be set up, in the absence and presence of an excess of a structurally distinct ligand, which also binds to the receptor of interest.
  - Binding that remains in the presence of an excess of the competing ligand is termed non-specific, whereas binding that is displaced is termed specific binding.

Saturation analysis

- Increasing the concentration of the labelled ligand leads to increased occupancy of the receptor (bound radioligand).
- At high concentrations of the labelled ligand, the receptor is fully occupied or saturated and so the shape of this binding curve is a rectangular hyperbola (Figure 5.12B).
- Binding of the labelled ligand to non-specific sites increases linearly with increasing concentration (Figure 5.12A).
- The graph of total binding (specific + non-specific binding) is therefore a combination of these two shapes, giving the appearance of a double rectangular hyperbola (Figure 5.12A).
- In practice, two parallel binding curves are generated and assessed: one has increasing concentrations of radioligand binding to the sample, while the second has exactly the same concentrations of radioligand binding to the sample in the presence of an excess of competing ligand (Figure 5.12A).
- Since the competing ligand prevents binding of the radioligand to the receptor, the difference between the two sets of data is the specific binding. This is calculated by simply subtracting the amount of radioligand bound in

the presence of competing ligand from the amount of radioligand bound in the absence of competing ligand (Figure 5.12B).

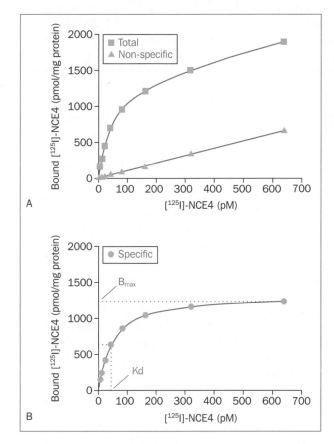

Figure 5.12 Saturation radioligand binding of [^{125}I]-NCE4 (novel chemical entity 4). A, Experimental data for binding of increasing concentrations of [^{125}I]-NCE4 in the absence (total) and presence (non-specific) of an excess of competing ligand. B, Specific binding of [^{125}I]-NCE4 (the numerical difference of total and non-specific binding) at increasing concentrations. Dashed lines allow definition of B_{max} and K_d values on the y- and x-axes, respectively.

- Ligand binding to the receptor is defined by the same equilibrium as we described earlier, albeit in a slightly different form:

$$L^* + R \rightleftharpoons L^*R$$

where L^* represents the ligand, R the free receptor and L^*R, the receptor–ligand complex. The equilibrium can be described with a dissociation constant, K_d:

$$K_d = \frac{[L^*][R]}{[L^*R]}$$

- Usually the K_d value is determined graphically from a saturation plot, since, by definition, the K_d value is equivalent to that concentration of radioligand which occupies 50% of the receptor. For most useful radioligands, the K_d value is between 10 pM and 10 nM.
- The B_{max}, also known as maximal binding capacity or receptor density, is the asymptote of binding or 100% specific binding and is also readily

determined graphically. For most tritiated radioligands, the useful lower limit of B_{max} values is about 100 fmol/mg protein, while radio-iodinated ligands can usefully measure binding levels down to 20 fmol/mg protein.

- In the example shown in Figure 5.12B, the B_{max} value for [^{125}I]-NCE4 binding is approximately 1300 fmol/mg protein, whereas the K_d value is approximately 40 pM.

Competition analysis

- Generating radiolabelled (or fluorescently tagged) versions of every drug to be assessed for binding affinity is laborious, expensive and impractical. Instead, it is possible to calculate binding affinities on the basis of competition for binding at the receptor with an established radioligand.
- A concentration of labelled ligand is used to achieve 'significant' occupancy of the receptor, usually between half and twice the K_d value. The concentration of radioligand employed may be influenced by the proportion of non-specific binding. For most useful radioligands, more than 50% of binding at about the K_d concentration of radioligand will be specific binding.
- Unlabelled ligands are co-incubated with the receptor source and radioligand over a range of concentrations, such that the unlabelled ligands compete for occupancy of the receptor by labelled ligand (bound radioligand).
- The shape of the resulting competition curve is sigmoidal or S-shaped, such that lowest concentrations of competing ligand fail to reduce bound radioligand, while the highest concentrations of competing ligand displace all the ligand bound to the receptor, so that bound levels are no different from non-specific binding (Figure 5.13).

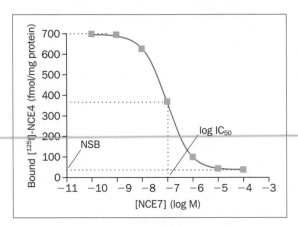

Figure 5.13 Competition analysis for [^{125}I]-NCE4 (novel chemical entity 4) binding using NCE7. NSB, non-specific binding.

- There are four useful parameters which may be obtained from non-linear analysis of a sigmoidal plot of the data (see above): the upper and lower asymptotes of binding, the concentration of competing ligand that displaces 50% of specific binding (IC$_{50}$ value) and the slope of the curve as it passes through the IC$_{50}$ point (expected to be −1 for a simple bimolecular interaction).

- The upper and lower asymptotes of the competition curve should coincide with levels of binding in the absence of competing ligand and non-specific binding, respectively (Figure 5.13). In this example, the upper asymptote is at 700, while the lower asymptote is at 40 fmol/mg protein. This allows calculation of the proportion of total binding which is to non-specific binding sites of 40/700 or approximately 6%. This ratio would make [125I]-NCE4 a useful radioligand to work with.
- The $\log IC_{50}$ and IC_{50} values of a competing ligand can vary with the level of radioligand occupancy of the receptor. This depends on:
  - radioligand affinity
  - radioligand concentration.
- Converting $\log IC_{50}$ and IC_{50} values to constants is enacted using the Cheng–Prusoff equation. To do this, both radioligand concentration and K_d value need to be obtained, the latter by prior saturation analysis. The constant derived by this equation is a K_i value (inhibitor dissociation constant):

$$K_i = \frac{IC_{50}}{1 + [RL]/K_d}$$

where $[RL]$ is the radioligand concentration and K_d is the radioligand dissociation constant. This may be rearranged to a logarithmic format to calculate pK_i values:

$$pK_i = pIC_{50} + \log\left(1 + [RL]/K_d\right)$$

- In the example shown in Figure 5.13, NCE7 competition for [125I]-NCE4 binding has a $\log IC_{50}$ of -7. Since [125I]-NCE4 was present at 40 pM, and the experiment illustrated in Figure 5.12B allowed estimation of the K_d value for [125I]-NCE4 binding of 40 pM, we can rapidly calculate the inhibitor dissociation constant for NCE7:

$$pK_i = 7 + \log\left(1 + 40/40\right) = 7 + \log(2) = 7 + 0.3 = 7.3$$

Alternatively,

$$K_i = \frac{1 \times 10^{-7}}{1 + 40/40} = \frac{1 \times 10^{-7}}{2} = 5 \times 10^{-8} M$$

- In some cases, the radioligand may bind to multiple sites or multiple affinity states of the same receptor (Figure 5.14). In this example, NCE7 displaces binding of the radioligand in two phases. A plateau is shown at 25% remaining bound radioligand where the concentration of NCE7 is sufficient to displace binding to a high-affinity site for NCE7, but is insufficient to displace binding to a low-affinity site for NCE7. In this example, therefore, 75% of radioligand is bound to a site which exhibits high affinity for NCE7, while 25% is bound to a low-affinity site for NCE7.

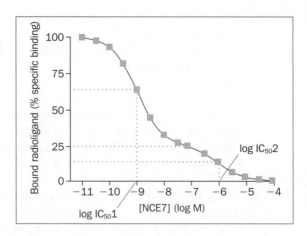

Figure 5.14 Biphasic competition curve. Novel chemical entity 7 (NCE7) discriminates two sites for [^{125}I]-NCE4 binding.

Determining the affinity of NCE7 for these two sites is conducted in two separate steps, using the Cheng–Prusoff equation described above.

■ For the NCE7 high-affinity site, where $\log IC_{50}1 = -9$:

$$pK_i = 9 + \log(1 + 40/40) = 9 + \log(2) = 9 + 0.3 = 9.3$$

■ For the NCE7 low-affinity site, where $\log IC_{50}2 = -6$:

$$pK_i = 6 + \log(1 + 40/40) = 6 + \log(2) = 6 + 0.3 = 6.3$$

■ Agonist competition for antagonist radioligand binding to a 7-transmembrane receptor (7TMR) is often (but not always) biphasic, because agonists exhibit high affinity for the G-protein-coupled form of the receptor and low affinity for the G-protein dissociated form (see Chapter 3). Antagonists do not discriminate between these two forms of the receptor, and so an antagonist radioligand saturation curve for binding to a 7TMR should be monophasic, i.e. there is only one binding site.

Kinetic parameters of radioligand binding

■ The binding parameters described above assume that binding has reached a steady state. That is, there is a dynamic equilibrium between radioligand binding to the receptor (providing an on-rate constant, k^{+1}) and radioligand dissociation from the receptor (off-rate constant, k^{-1}). At steady state, these two actions are balanced.

■ It is also possible to obtain useful data using a kinetic approach for radioligand binding, since the ratio of on-rate and off-rate constants is equivalent to the affinity constant.

$$L^* + R \underset{k^{-1}}{\overset{k^{+1}}{\rightleftharpoons}} L^*R$$

■ To determine the off-rate constant, radioligand binding is allowed to take place until steady state is reached and then an excess of competing ligand is added. This excess of competing ligand ensures that, as radioligand dissociates from the receptor, the possibility of radioligand once more binding to the receptor is infinitesimally small, so that the only influence on the amount of radioligand bound is the off-rate (k^{-1}). Diluting the incubation in a large volume of buffer (at least 100-fold) allows an off-rate constant to be measured through a similar process.

■ Since this is an exponential rate, it can be determined graphically using the natural log of bound radioligand against time. However, computer programs allow iterative non-linear fitting of exponential curves to such data to calculate k^{-1} (Figure 5.15). In the example shown in Figure 5.15, the rate of radioligand dissociation is assessed at three concentrations of radioligand, [^{3}H]-NCE14, equivalent to well below the K_d concentration (0.25 nM), close to the K_d concentration (1 nM) and well in excess of the K_d concentration (4 nM). At the highest concentration of radioligand, the determined half-life of dissociation $(t_{1/2})$ is quickest.

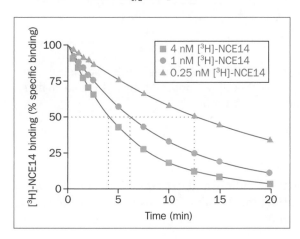

Figure 5.15 Dissociation kinetic analysis of radioligand binding. Binding in the presence of three different concentrations of radioligand was allowed to reach steady state, before dissociation of radioligand was initiated in the presence of an excess of competing ligand. Note that half-times for dissociation increase with decreasing radioligand concentration.

■ The dissociation rate constant is then calculated from the following relationship:

$$k^{-1} = 0.69/t_{1/2}$$

■ Units of the dissociation rate constant are in inverse time units, usually 1/min. For the example shown in Figure 5.15, the half-times were estimated to be 4.1, 6.2 and 12.8 min for radioligand concentrations of 4, 1 and 0.25 nM [^{3}H]-NCE14, respectively. From these data, k^{-1} values of 0.17, 0.11 and 0.054/min can be calculated.

■ To determine the on-rate, binding is allowed to take place with frequent sampling of levels of bound radioligand until a steady state is reached (Figure 5.16). In the example shown in Figure 5.16, using the same three concentrations of radioligand employed in the determination of radioligand off-rate, it can be seen that binding occurs more rapidly with higher concentrations.

- From the example shown in Figure 5.16, half-times to steady state are 0.69, 2.8 and 9.7 min for 4, 1 and 0.25 nM [³H]-NCE14, respectively. From these, we can calculate values for k_{obs} of 1, 0.25 and 0.071/min, respectively.

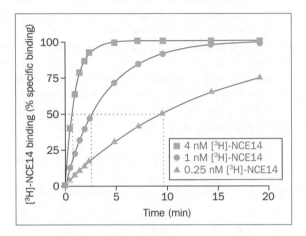

Figure 5.16 Association kinetic analysis of radioligand binding. Note that half-times for apparent association decrease with increasing radioligand concentration.

- Since radioligand is also dissociating from the receptor at the same time, the rate observed, k_{obs}, is a composite of both on- and off-rates, as well as being influenced by the radioligand concentration.

$$k^{+1} = \frac{k_{obs} - k^{-1}}{[RL]}$$

- Calculated k^{+1} values for the three radioligand concentrations are 0.21, 0.14 and 0.066/min/nM. By definition, the K_d value is equivalent to the ratio of the off-rate divided by the on-rate, or:

$$K_d = \frac{k^{-1}}{k^{+1}}$$

- For the three concentrations, therefore:

$$K_d^{4\,nM} = \frac{0.169}{0.21} = 0.80 \; nM$$

$$K_d^{1\,nM} = \frac{0.11}{0.14} = 0.79 \; nM$$

$$K_d^{0\,nM} = \frac{0.054}{0.066} = 0.82 \; nM$$

- As expected, kinetic experiments give very similar estimates of K_d values at all three concentrations of radioligand.

Distinguishing a binding site from a receptor

- In order to define a binding site as a particular receptor, binding must be saturable, reflective of a limited number of receptors in a given tissue.
- With the exception noted above, for agonist competition for antagonist radioligand binding to 7TMR, binding should be monophasic (to a single site).
- Binding should be specific, with quantitative binding parameters commensurate with established pharmacology for the receptor.
- The localisation of binding to tissue and subcellular fractions should correlate with functional responses evoked by that receptor.

Applications of radioligand binding

- It is useful in determining changes in receptor number, investigating changes following chronic drug treatments or denervation.
- With the refinement of autoradiography, radioligand binding allows cellular and, occasionally, subcellular localisation of the receptor to be assessed. This may allow hypotheses to be constructed as to physiological roles of the receptor.
- Radioligand binding may be employed to check receptor levels during protein isolation procedures or for identifying clonal cell lines expressing recombinant receptor.
- It has also been employed for identifying novel endogenous ligands of receptors.
- The most frequent applications, however, are in the identification of receptor mechanisms and in novel drug discovery.

Enzyme–substrate and transporter–substrate interactions

- The quantification of substrate interaction with either enzymes or transporters is based on the measurement of rates of substrate conversion to product or substrate accumulation, respectively, using a Michaelis–Menten plot (Figure 5.17).

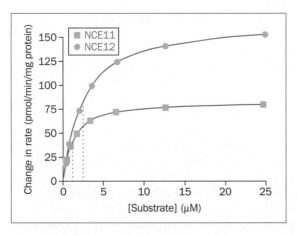

Figure 5.17 Michaelis–Menten plot of enzyme–substrate (or transporter–substrate) interactions. For the data illustrated, novel chemical entity 11 (NCE11) exhibits a K_m value of 1 µM, while NCE10 has a K_m value of 2.3 µM. V_{max} values for the two substrates are 80 and 160 pmol/min/mg protein, respectively.

- Plotting rates of substrate conversion or accumulation against increasing concentrations of substrate generates a rectangular hyperbola.
- In the examples shown in Figure 5.17, the two substrates exhibit distinct substrate affinities (K_m) and maximal rates (V_{max}), which may be determined in exactly the same manner as binding parameters of a radioligand.
- NCE10 has a V_{max} of 150 pmol/min/mg protein with a K_m of 2.5 µM. In comparison, NCE11 has a lower maximal rate (a V_{max} of 75 pmol/min/mg protein) with a higher affinity (a K_m of 1 µM).

Assessing the effects of inhibitors

- The affinity of inhibitors is normally assessed by the use of a fixed concentration of inhibitor with a range of substrate concentrations.
- Traditionally, these were analysed by conversion to plots which allow linear regression to be conducted. The Lineweaver–Burk (or double reciprocal) and Eadie–Hofstee plots have mostly been replaced with the availability of computer programs able to conduct iterative non-linear regression.
- These allow identification of inhibitor affinity, as well as allowing interpretation of the mode of action of the inhibitor.
- Inhibitors which increase solely the substrate affinity, K_m, are competitive, while agents which inhibit solely the maximal rate, V_{max}, are non-competitive.
- Inhibitors which alter both K_m and V_{max} values may be either mixed inhibitors or, more rarely, uncompetitive inhibitors.
- One of the few examples of uncompetitive inhibitors is lithium ion inhibition of inositol monophosphatase activity. This is significant because uncompetitive inhibitors have little effect at low substrate concentrations, but impede the rate of conversion (or transport) at high substrate concentrations, meaning that only the most active cells will show significant effects of the inhibitor.

Drug selectivity and target identification

- What constitutes a specific or selective drug?
- A specific drug is one which only acts at a single target, without the involvement of any other target.
- Very few, if any, drugs in clinical usage match this criterion.
- A 'good' drug for defining the involvement of a particular target would be one which has 1000-fold selectivity for the target of interest (for example, an agent with a K_i value of 1 nM at the receptor of interest, with pK_i values of greater than 1 µM at every other receptor, would be a useful agent in pharmacological, and potentially clinical, situations).
- Not many therapeutic agents are this selective. For example, the majority of β_1-adrenoceptor-selective antagonists in clinical usage show a selectivity ratio for β_1- versus β_2-adrenoceptors of 20-fold or less.
- As there are so few drugs available with 1000-fold selectivity ratios for pharmacological targets, but frequently a number of drugs with a range of selectivities and a range of affinities, the preferred means of identifying the

involvement of a particular drug target is to use multiple agents (preferably antagonists or inhibitors) to construct a rank order of affinities to compare with established values (usually derived from investigations of recombinant proteins).

■ One useful way of conducting such analysis is to perform linear correlation, comparing estimates of ligand affinity in the experimental situation with those at recombinant receptors, transporters or enzyme.

KeyPoint

■ Quantitative description of drug effects is crucial to predicting their selectivity and clinical efficacy.

chapter 6
Autonomic pharmacology

Organisation of the autonomic nervous system

- The autonomic nervous system (ANS) carries the output of the central nervous system to all peripheral organs except voluntary muscle. It influences all of the body's activities that do not require conscious control, e.g. heart rate, breathing, digestion.
- It is organised anatomically and functionally into sympathetic and parasympathetic divisions.
- Both divisions consist of networks comprising two neurones in series (Figure 6.1); the first neurone (preganglionic) in both divisions releases acetylcholine (ACh) which activates nicotinic receptors (ACh-gated cation channels) located on the second (postganglionic) neurone's cell body.

Figure 6.1 The organisation of the autonomic nervous system. ACh, acetylcholine; NA, noradrenaline.

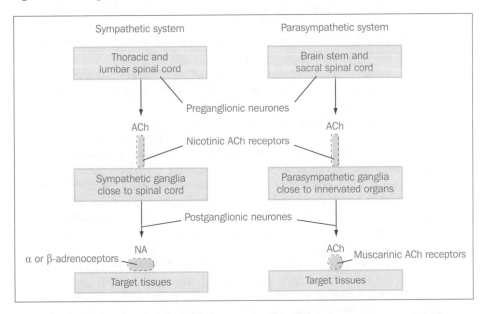

- The cell bodies of postganglionic neurones are located in ganglia, close to the spinal cord, in the case of the sympathetic division, or close to the innervated target tissues in the case of the parasympathetic division.
- The neurotransmitter released from postganglionic neurones in the sympathetic system is usually noradrenaline (NA), which activates α- or β-adrenoceptors on target cells.

- An exception to this is the sweat glands, the innervation of which is anatomically and functionally sympathetic but, in this case, the postganglionic neurone releases ACh to activate muscarinic receptors on the glands.
- Another exception to the general rule is the adrenal gland where a single neurone releases ACh to activate nicotinic receptors on the adrenal medulla, causing the release of adrenaline into the circulation. In this case the adrenal medulla plays the role of a typical sympathetic postganglionic neurone (stimulated by ACh and releasing a catecholamine).
- The neurotransmitter released from postganglionic parasympathetic neurones is ACh, which activates muscarinic receptors on target cells.
- Functionally, the sympathetic system prepares the body for physical activity (the famous fight or flight reflex) whilst the parasympathetic system primes for feeding and relaxation.
- Muscarinic ACh receptors and α-adrenoceptors generally cause contraction and β-adrenoceptors cause relaxation of the smooth muscle present in many target organs.
- Blood vessels have very little parasympathetic innervation. Sympathetic stimulation generally causes constriction, via β-adrenoceptors, of arterioles and veins and dilatation (arterioles in voluntary muscle and veins) via β-adrenoceptors.
- The heart (cardiac muscle force and rate of contraction) is excited by sympathetically activated β_1-adrenoceptors and inhibited by parasympathetically activated muscarinic receptors.
- Bronchial smooth muscle is contracted by ACh (muscarinic receptors) and relaxed by noradrenaline (β_2-adrenoceptors).
- In the gut, motility is decreased by the sympathetic system (combination of α- and β_2-adrenoceptors) and increased by the parasympathetic system (muscarinic receptors) which also increase secretions. Sphincters are constricted sympathetically and relaxed parasympathetically.
- In the eye, the pupil size is increased due to sympathetic (α-adrenoceptors) constriction of the radial smooth muscle (dilator pupillae) and reduced due to the parasympathetic (muscarinic) constriction of the circular smooth muscle (constrictor pupillae). Focusing for near vision is achieved by parasympathetic contraction of the ciliary muscle, which allows the lens to bulge.
- In the penis, erection is parasympathetic but ejaculation is sympathetic.
- The sympathetic system alone controls glucose synthesis and liberation from glycogen in the liver.
- In addition to the 'traditional' neurotransmitters, ACh and noradrenaline, there are a number of non-adrenergic, non-cholinergic (NANC) transmitters used by the ANS. The major ones are adenosine triphosphate (ATP) and neuropeptide Y (NPY) in the sympathetic system and nitric oxide and vasointestinal polypeptide (VIP) in the parasympathetic system. These may be co-released with noradrenaline or ACh.
- The release of neurotransmitters from ANS nerve endings can be controlled by presynaptic receptors. For example, noradrenaline released from a sympathetic terminal could act on α_2-adrenoceptors located on adjoining parasympathetic terminals to reduce ACh release. These α_2-adrenoceptors

would be referred to as heteroceptors as they control the release of a transmitter different from the one they exist to recognise. If presynaptic α_2-adrenoceptors limited noradrenaline release from a sympathetic terminal they would be referred to as autoreceptors because they would be controlling the release of a transmitter which they recognise.

- The mechanism of control of transmitter release is mainly through the modulation of calcium and potassium channels. Activation of calcium channels increases release; activation of potassium channels decreases release.
- Postsynaptic modulation of the effects of ANS transmitters is also possible. For example, NPY is co-released with noradrenaline from some sympathetic terminals and enhances blood vessel constriction.
- The pre- and postsynaptic modification of responses is referred to as neuromodulation.
- The termination of autonomic neurotransmitter action can either be by rapid metabolism, as in the case of ACh by the enzyme acetylcholine esterase, or by reuptake into surrounding cells in the case of noradrenaline.

Pharmacology of the autonomic nervous system

Acetylcholine receptors
- Nicotinic receptors are found in neuromuscular junctions and in all autonomic ganglia. These ACh-activated cation channels differ somewhat in structure and, therefore, pharmacology (see Chapter 27). ACh and nicotine (hence the name) are agonists at both neuromuscular junction and neuronal nicotinic receptors.
- Nicotinic receptor agonists are used in smoking cessation.
- Nicotinic receptor antagonists selective for the neuronal channels (hexamethonium, trimetaphan) inhibit transmission at all autonomic ganglia and, hence, are referred to as ganglion-blocking drugs. Ganglion blockade could also be achieved by inhibiting preganglionic ACh release (e.g. with the bacterial poison botulinum toxin). The effects of ganglion blockade are many and varied given the indiscriminate inhibition of both ANS divisions. The most important effects are cardiovascular with the inhibition of all reflexes leading to reduced arterial blood pressure and postural hypotension (fainting on standing up). There are no longer any therapeutic indications for ganglion-blocking drugs.
- Muscarinic receptors are G-protein-coupled receptors (see Chapter 3). There are five subtypes, three of which (M_1, M_3, M_5) are Ca^{2+}-mobilising receptors ($G_{q/11}$-linked) and the others (M_2, M_4) inhibit cyclic adenosine monophosphate (AMP) formation (G_i-linked). In relation to the ANS, M_1 receptors are found in the stomach and salivary glands where they increase secretions. There are also some M_1 receptors in the autonomic ganglia where they potentiate the mainly nicotinic effects of ACh. M_2 receptors are located in the heart where they mediate reduction in rate and force of contraction. M_3 receptors increase secretion from endocrine and exocrine glands, contract smooth muscle (e.g. pupillary muscle) but mediate vasorelaxation (indirectly through nitric oxide formation).

- There are few therapeutic uses for muscarinic receptor agonists, although pilocarpine (in eye drops) is used as a miotic (reduces pupil diameter) which relieves raised intraocular pressure in closed-angle glaucoma by freeing up the drainage of aqueous humour. It is also used rarely for treating dry mouth after radiation treatment. Such actions are referred to as parasympathomimetic since they mimic effects of parasympathetic system activation.
- There are a variety of subtype-selective muscarinic receptor antagonists but all subtypes are blocked by atropine. The M_1-selective antagonist pirenzepine was used as a gastric ulcer treatment but has been withdrawn. The non-selective antagonist ipratropium bromide relaxes airway smooth muscle and is used as an inhalation therapy in asthma and chronic obstructive pulmonary disease (see Chapter 17). Atropine, tropicamide and the longer-acting cyclopentolate are used topically to increase pupil diameter (mydriasis) to facilitate ophthalmic examination.
- Muscarinic antagonists like atropine, given systemically, would reduce the effects of the parasympathetic system leading to inhibition of secretions (e.g. dry mouth), tachycardia, relaxation of smooth muscle (gut, airways, bladder), pupillary dilatation and paralysis of accommodation.

Acetylcholinesterase

- The action of ACh is terminated by rapid catabolism (to choline and acetate) by cholinesterases. Acetylcholinesterase (AChE) is selective for ACh catabolism and is bound to cholinergic synaptic membranes, where its task is to break down released ACh, and in a soluble form in cholinergic terminals where it regulates free ACh levels.
- Inhibition of AChE, therefore, preserves ACh and potentiates its effects at the neuromuscular junction, autonomic ganglia, in the central nervous system and parasympathetic target tissues.
- AChE inhibitors can be short-acting (e.g. edrophonium), medium-acting (e.g. neostigmine) or irreversible (organophosphates such as ecothiopate). Some nerve gases and insecticides are long-acting AChE inhibitors.
- Autonomic effects of the inhibitors include excessive secretions, hypotension, bradycardia, gut hypermotility and bronchoconstriction.
- Clinical uses include diagnosis and treatment of myasthenia gravis (autoimmune destruction of neuromuscular joint nicotinic receptors leading to muscle weakness) and in anaesthesia as an antidote to non-depolarising neuromuscular blockers (see Chapter 27). Interestingly, the muscarinic side-effects wear off relatively rapidly (receptor desensitisation?). Ecothiopate was formerly used as a local miotic treatment for glaucoma.

Adrenoceptors

- These are G-protein-coupled receptors (see Chapter 3) which are categorised into three major subgroups (Table 6.1):
  1. α_1-adrenoceptors, which are Ca^{2+}-mobilising ($G_{q/11}$-linked) receptors
  2. α_2-adrenoceptors, which inhibit cyclic AMP via G_i
  3. β-adrenoceptors, which increase cyclic AMP via G_s proteins.

Table 6.1 Selective agonists and antagonists of adrenoceptors

	α_1-adrenoceptor	α_2-adrenoceptor	β_1-adrenoceptor	β_2-adrenoceptor	β_3-adrenoceptor
Selective agonist	Phenylephrine	Clonidine	Xamoterol	Salbutamol Salmeterol	Carazolol
Selective antagonist	Prazosin	Rauwolscine	Atenolol Betaxolol	ICI 118551	SR59230A

- α_1-adrenoceptors mediate smooth-muscle contraction; α_2-adrenoceptors also cause contraction of smooth muscle and inhibition of neurotransmitter release. The β_1 subtype causes heart muscle contraction and the β_2 subtype causes airway smooth-muscle relaxation. A third β-adrenoceptor subtype, β_3, enhances lipolysis.
- The endogenous agonists noradrenaline and adrenaline stimulate all adrenoceptors, albeit with somewhat different potencies.

Clinical uses of adrenoceptor ligands

- Phenylephrine is used in eye drops as a mydriatic agent for ophthalmic examination and by injection/infusion for acute hypotension.
- Prazosin is antihypertensive; it can cause collapse due to severe hypotension (see Chapter 13).
- Clonidine acts centrally to reduce blood pressure and can be used in migraine and menopausal flushing.
- Beta-blockers such as betaxolol are used to reduce intraocular pressure in glaucoma (see Chapter 13 for uses in cardiovascular disease).
- β_2-adrenoceptor agonists are used as bronchodilators in asthma (see Chapter 17).

Indirectly acting sympathomimetic drugs

- Adrenoceptor agonists can be referred to as directly acting sympathomimetics because they mimic the action of noradrenaline released from sympathetic nerves. Indirectly acting sympathomimetic agents such as tyramine, ephedrine and amphetamine are sufficiently like noradrenaline to be taken up into nerve terminals where they displace the natural transmitter which is then released passively into the synapse (i.e. not by exocytosis).
- Ephedrine is used as a nasal decongestant but excessive use causes rebound congestion. Amphetamine has marked central nervous system effects (see Chapter 25).
- The enzyme monoamine oxidase metabolises noradrenaline and controls its levels in sympathetic terminals but has no influence on released transmitter. Monoamine oxidase inhibitors (see Chapter 20) do not, therefore, have a major sympathomimetic action although they do markedly potentiate the effects of indirectly acting sympathomimetics such as tyramine.

Uptake inhibitors

- The actions of noradrenaline are terminated by uptake into surrounding cells by selective transporter proteins. Inhibition by tricyclic antidepressants (e.g. imipramine; see Chapter 20) or cocaine (see Chapter 25) enhances the effects of released noradrenaline, leading to mainly central but also some peripheral effects (e.g. tachycardia).

Other drugs acting on sympathetic nerve terminals

- So-called noradrenergic neurone-blocking drugs, e.g. guanethidine, are transported into sympathetic terminals and concentrated in vesicles where they prevent noradrenaline release by a local anaesthetic-like action. They very effectively reduce blood pressure and were used in the past as antihypertensives, but they abolish all sympathetic tone and reflexes, leading to unacceptable side-effects such as postural hypotension and diarrhoea.
- Reserpine prevents the accumulation of noradrenaline in vesicles, eventually leading to its depletion and reduced sympathetic tone. It reduces blood pressure, but leads to severe depression via monoamine transmitter depletion in the brain.

Key Points

- To a large extent, the sympathetic and parasympathetic divisions of the ANS oppose each other's actions.
- The sympathetic system prepares for 'fight or flight' and the parasympathetic system for feeding and relaxation.
- ACh acting on nicotinic receptors is the neurotransmitter at all autonomic ganglia.
- The main sympathetic postganglionic neurotransmitter is noradrenaline, which stimulates α- and β-adrenoceptors on target tissues.
- The main parasympathetic postganglionic neurotransmitter is ACh, which stimulates muscarinic receptors on target tissues.
- Other NANC transmitters exist in the ANS and these can be co-released with noradrenaline and ACh.
- The action of released ACh is terminated by AChE.
- The action of released noradrenaline is terminated by reuptake.
- Parasympathomimetic effects can be brought about directly by muscarinic receptor agonists and indirectly by AChE inhibitors.
- Sympathomimetic effects can be brought about directly by α- and β-adrenoceptor agonists and indirectly by noradrenaline displacers such as ephedrine or reuptake inhibitors.

Self-assessment

1. **Fill in the missing words:**
a. The neurotransmitter released by all preganglionic autonomic neurones is

_____ .

b. The receptors for ACh on all postganglionic autonomic neurones are of the
_____ type.
_____ is the neurotransmitter released by most postganglionic
sympathetic neurones.
c. The receptors for ACh on most tissues innervated by the parasympathetic
system are of the _____ type.

2. **Answer true or false to the following statements:**
a. If an α_2-adrenoceptor mediates the reduction of noradrenaline release from a
sympathetic neurone it should be referred to as an autoreceptor.
b. Noradrenaline and ACh are the only neurotransmitters employed by the
ANS.
c. ATP and NPY are co-transmitters in the parasympathetic system.
d. The action of released noradrenaline is terminated by the enzyme
monoamine oxidase.

3. **Fill in the missing words:**
a. Blood vessels have very little _____ innervation.
b. Gut motility is increased by activation of the _____ division of the
ANS.
c. Bronchial smooth muscle is relaxed by _____ and contracted by

_____ .

d. Blockade of muscarinic receptors in the pupillary smooth muscle causes
_____ of the pupil.

4. **Which of the following effects would be expected to follow treatment with
an acetylcholine esterase inhibitor?**
a. Hypotension with bradycardia
b. Reduced gut motility
c. Mydriasis
d. Bronchoconstriction

5. **Fill in the missing words:**
a. Prazosin is a selective antagonist of _____ .
b. Ephedrine is an _____ sympathomimetic drug.
c. α_1-adrenoceptors are linked to the _____ protein and cause
_____ mobilisation.
d. β_2-adrenoceptor agonists (e.g. salbutamol) are used in the treatment of
_____ because they cause _____ .

chapter 7
Local mediators

In contrast to hormones, which are released into the blood stream to act at a remote site, local mediators act on the cells from which they were released (autocrine function) or on immediately adjacent cells (paracrine function).

Histamine

- Histamine is synthesised by histidine decarboxylase, an enzyme found primarily in mast cells and nervous tissue.
- Histamine appears to function as a stimulus for bone resorption.
- It is primarily associated with mast cells or basophils and plays a role in the acute immune response. The primary stimulus for mast cell degranulation is activation of immunoglobulin E (IgE) receptors on the cell surface. The histamine released acts on H_1 receptors to increase blood flow and sensitise primary afferent nerves and capillary permeability. In the lung, released histamine causes bronchoconstriction through H_1 receptors, which are targets for antihistamines used in the treatment of hayfever and allergen sensitivities.

Gasotransmitters

Although there are many similarities with conventional transmitters (regulated biosynthesis, well-defined and specific functions at physiologically relevant concentrations through specific cellular and molecular targets), gasotransmitters differ in that they are small gaseous molecules, freely permeable to membranes and, hence, made on demand.

Nitric oxide

Nitric oxide (NO) is the archetypal gasotransmitter, but recently two further gases, carbon monoxide and hydrogen sulphide, have been described to fit the above criteria for definition as gasotransmitters. Ammonia, sulphur dioxide and nitrous oxide are three further gasotransmitter candidates.

NO (a gaseous radical) has a role as a neurotransmitter in the gastrointestinal tract, but is best characterised physiologically as a regulator of vascular tone. This classical role can be defined as a sequence of events.

Activation of endothelial G_q-coupled receptors (see Chapter 3), e.g. substance P (NK_1), receptors leads to the following sequence of events:

- activation of phospholipase C, leading to generation of inositol 1,4,5-trisphosphate and elevation of intracellular calcium levels
- stimulation of the endothelial form of NO synthase and the subsequent generation of NO

- diffusion of NO
- activation of soluble guanylyl cyclase and the generation of 3',5'-cyclic guanosine monophosphate (cGMP) in the adjacent smooth-muscle cells
- activation of cGMP-dependent protein kinase (PKG)
- phosphorylation and inhibition of myosin light-chain kinase
- vasorelaxation.

Although NO is not stored as such, there are roles for carrier molecules, which may allow for either longer-lasting responses to stimuli or action at more remote targets.

- NO reacts reversibly with thiols to form nitrosothiols (e.g. S-nitrosoglutathione: GSNO):
  - potential intracellular carrier function?
- NO also reacts reversibly with oxyhaemoglobin in circulating erythrocytes:
  - potential extracellular carrier function?

The vasorelaxatant role of NO is mimicked by nitrovasodilators, such as glyceryl trinitrate and isosorbide dinitrate, used in the treatment of angina pectoris to increase blood flow through the coronary vessels. Nitrergic (i.e. NO-mediated) transmission is amplified through the use of phosphodiesterase 5 (PDE_5) inhibitors, such as sildenafil and vardenafil, in the treatment of male erectile dysfunction.

A distinct, inducible form of NO synthase is found in cells of the immune system in response to pathogens. The NO generated by this route not only causes local vasodilatation, but also sensitises primary afferent nerves and results in nitrosylation of:

- lipids (e.g. nitrolinoleate)
- proteins (nitrotyrosine)
- DNA
  - leading to indiscriminate damage, to host and to the pathogen.

Eicosanoids

Eicosanoids are a family of more than 40 metabolites, largely derived from the oxidative metabolism of arachidonic acid, with about 25 receptors, primarily 7-transmembrane receptors (7TMRs), but also nuclear receptors and transmitter-gated channels.

- includes multiple entities with complex interconversion:
  - prostanoids, leukotrienes, epoxyeicosatrienoic acids (EETs), endocannabinoids, resolvins, lipoxins (LXs), isoprostanes
- no storage
- made on demand
- 7TMRs
  - 9 prostanoid receptors
  - 4 leukotriene receptors
  - 1/2 LX receptors
  - 1 oxoeicosatrienoic acid (OXE) receptor

- 1 ResolvinE1 (RvE1) receptor
- 2/3 cannabinoid receptors
- 4 free fatty acid (FFA) receptors
■ nuclear receptors
- 3 peroxisome proliferator-activated receptor (PPARs)
■ transmitter-gated channels
- 2 transient receptor potential (TRP) receptors
■ 30+ enzymes.

Arachidonic acid generation

Arachidonic acid is thought to be generated primarily through the action of a family of enzymes, termed phospholipase A_2 (PLA$_2$), which hydrolyses the major membrane phospholipid phosphatidylcholine, producing lysophosphatidylcholine as a byproduct.

■ PLA$_2$ isoforms are ubiquitous.
■ cPLA$_2$ isoforms are activated downstream of a wide variety of stimuli:
- elevated intracellular free calcium ions (i.e. > 100 nM):
  Ca^{2+} mobilisation by Gq-coupled 7TMRs
  Ca^{2+}-gating receptors, such as N-methyl-D-aspartate (NMDA) glutamate receptors
  depolarisation-evoked calcium entry through voltage-sensitive calcium channels
- phosphorylation (protein kinase C, mitogen-activated protein kinase)
- Gβγ subunits from heterotrimeric G-proteins
■ Upon activation, translocates from the cytosol to the plasma membrane.
■ No selective inhibitors of PLA$_2$ exist.
■ The arachidonic acid released can be metabolised through three major oxidative routes: epoxygenases, lipoxygenases and/or cyclooxygenases (COX).

Epoxygenases and EETs

■ CYP450-like enzyme/s (CYP2C/J?) active at any of the four double bonds of arachidonic acid
■ Produces EETs:
- EETs are vasorelaxant through undefined targets
- open K^+ channels causing hyperpolarisation
- metabolised by epoxide hydrolase.
■ Relatively selective inhibitors of epoxygenase and soluble epoxide hydrolase activities have been described, although these are of pharmacological interest rather than of therapeutic value.

Lipoxygenases, leukotrienes and lipoxins

■ 5-Lipoxygenase (5-LOX) is predominantly expressed in leukocytes.
■ Oxidation and rearrangement via a two-step reaction of 5-LOX activity produces 5-hydroperoxyeicosatetraenoic acid (5-HPETE) and leukotriene A_4 (LTA$_4$), giving rise to the classically defined slow-releasing substance of anaphylaxis (SRS-A).

- 5-LOX is activated by:
  - FLAP (5-lipoxygenase-activating protein)
  - elevated $[Ca^{2+}]_i$ (i.e. > 100 nM)
  - mitogen-activated protein kinases.
- It is inhibited by cyclic AMP-dependent protein kinase.
- The LTA_4 produced can be converted by a specific hydrolase to LTB_4 or conjugated to glutathione to form the cysteinyl leukotrienes, LTC_4 and LTD_4.
- LTB_4 activates BLT_1 and BLT_2 receptors, while LTC_4 and LTD_4 activate $CysLT_1$ and $CysLT_2$ receptors.
- All four of these receptors are G_q-coupled 7TMRs and at least two of them are expressed on leukocytes and bronchial smooth muscle.
- Given that both PLA_2 and 5-LOX activity may be activated by G_q-coupled receptors, this provides a mechanism whereby a rapid anaphylactic response can be elicited involving a major amplification of leukotriene generation and, hence, bronchoconstriction.
- Zileuton and montelukast are examples of medicines which inhibit 5-LOX and $CysLT_1$ receptors, respectively. They are used prophylactically for the treatment of hayfever and childhood asthma (see Chapters 17 and 18).

Transcellular metabolism of leukotrienes

- Studies of LTA_4 incubation with platelets identified LXs.
- Sequential leukocyte 5-LOX and platelet 12/15-LOX generates LXA_4.
- These are agonists at ALX LX receptors, which have an anti-inflammatory profile and may represent a 'stop' signal for inflammation.
- Given that platelets adhere to leukocytes in inflammatory conditions, the transcellular metabolism of arachidonic acid represents a significant therapeutic opportunity.

Leukotriene–LX interactions

- 5-LOX:
  - metabolises arachidonic acid to produce LTs
  - also metabolises 15-HETE to produce LXs
- 15-LOX:
  - metabolises arachidonic acid to produce 15-HETE
  - ~~also metabolises LTs to produce LXs~~
- LXA_4:
  - high-potency full agonist at ALX receptors
  - low-potency partial agonist at $CysLT_1$ receptors
- LTC_4:
  - high-potency full agonist at $CysLT_1$ receptors
  - low-potency partial agonist at ALX receptors
- The presence of the distinct blood particles and the interlocking pathways they represent, therefore, allows a balance between pro- and anti-inflammatory signals.

Cyclooxygenase activity and prostanoids

One of two COX enzymes, which are widely distributed, generating prostaglandin (PG) H_2, COX-1 is generally considered to be constitutively active, producing metabolites evoking physiological responses. In contrast, COX-2 activity is thought to produce metabolites involved in pathological conditions. Depending on the cell type, further metabolism generates distinct prostanoids.

- PGD_2 synthase, highly expressed in mast cells, generates PGD_2.
- PGE_2 synthase, highly expressed in macrophages and fibroblasts, generates PGE_2.
- $PGF_{2\alpha}$ synthase, suggested to be prominently expressed in the uterus and in the eye, generates $PGF_{2\alpha}$.
- PGI_2 synthase, highly expressed in the vascular endothelium, generates prostacyclin.
- Thromboxane A_2 (TxA_2) synthase, a cytochrome P450 enzyme highly expressed in platelets, generates TxA_2.

Prostanoid turnover

- PGs are exported from cells by membrane transporters (apparently the multidrug resistance protein 4, MRP4, also known as ABCC4).
- PGs are accumulated in cells by a PG transporter.
- Intracellular PGs are metabolised by 15-hydroxyprostaglandin dehydrogenase:
  - ubiquitous enzyme
  - generates 15-ketoprostanoids, which are much lower-potency ligands at prostanoid receptors.
- TxA_2 is also hydrolysed at epoxide to produce lower-potency TxB_2.

The prostanoids generated have activity at numerous sites in the body:
- They are agonists at 7TMRs:
  - four G_q-coupled receptors (EP_1, EP_3, FP and TP receptors)
  - four G_s-coupled receptors (EP_2, EP_4, DP_1 and IP receptors)
  - one G_i-coupled receptor (DP_2 receptors)
- They regulate smooth-muscle contractility:
  - IP receptors, activated by prostacyclin, are relaxatory.
  - FP and TP receptors, activated by $PGF_{2\alpha}$ and TxA_2, are contractile.
- Platelet function:
  - TP and DP_2 receptors are proaggregatory.
  - IP receptors are antiaggregatory.

Inhibitors of prostanoid action

- COX inhibitors:
  - Non-steroidal anti-inflammatory drugs (aspirin, indometacin, ibuprofen, diclofenac, naproxen)
    analgesics, antipyretics and anti-inflammatories to differing extents
    the reduction in prostanoid generation reduces sensitisation of primary afferent nerves, reduces activation of hypothalamic nerves and reduces recruitment of elements of the immune system

- COX-2 inhibitors (celecoxib)
  therapies for chronic inflammatory conditions
- PG receptor antagonists
  - TP/DP$_2$ (ramatroban)
    coronary artery disease and asthma.

Endocannabinoids/endovanilloids

These are ester or amide analogues of arachidonic acid, with the 'best' candidate for the endogenous agonist of cannabinoid receptors being the ester 2-arachidonoylglycerol.

- two cannabinoid G-protein-coupled receptors (CB$_1$ and CB$_2$)
- both G$_{i/o}$-coupled receptors
- CB$_1$ highest-density 7TMRs in the central nervous system (2 pmol/mg protein)
  - elicits inhibition of transmitter release
- CB$_2$ primarily associated with immune system.

Anandamide, an amide of arachidonic acid, although exhibiting agonist activity at cannabinoid receptors, is a better candidate for the endogenous agonist of TRPV1 vanilloid receptors.

- TRPV1 (VR1/capsaicin receptor) gates Ca^{2+}
- activated by low pH, noxious heat (>43°C)
- predominantly expressed in a subset of primary afferent neurones
- mediates burning sensation of hot chilli peppers.

Given that anandamide is generated through intracellular routes and the binding site for TRPV1 activation is also intracellular, anandamide represents a potential intracrine ligand. It has been proposed that chronic pain states are associated with a balance between (amongst other influences) activation of pro-nociceptive TRPV1 receptors and anti-nociceptive CB$_1$ and CB$_2$ receptors.

KeyPoints

- Local mediators are not stored, but rather are made on demand.
- They act on cells in the immediate vicinity to elicit responses.

Self-assessment

Fill in the gaps in the following sentences:

1. Nitric oxide is generated by the enzyme nitric oxide _____.
2. Nitric oxide activates the enzyme _____ guanylyl cyclase.
3. Arachidonic acid is found in the _____ position of most membrane phospholipids.
4. Cytochrome P450-like enzymes metabolise arachidonic acid to form _____.
5. 5-Lipoxygenase activity can be inhibited by _____.
6. Leukotriene A_4 is generated by _____ activity.
7. Montelukast blocks _____ receptors.
8. LXA_4 is a full agonist at _____ LX receptors.
9. COX activity converts arachidonic acid to _____.
10. PGs are inactivated by the enzyme _____.

chapter 8
Pharmacokinetics and drug metabolism

Pharmacokinetics and drug metabolism refer to how the body handles a drug from absorption, distribution, and metabolism to excretion (ADME).

Absorption and bioavailability (*F*)

- Intravenous administration leads to 100% of a drug entering the body. The oral route may lead to slower and incomplete absorption.

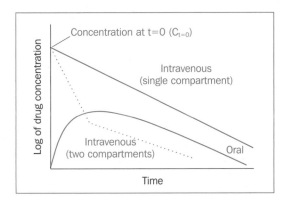

Figure 8.1 A concentration–time plot for oral and intravenous drug administration. The intravenous plot is given for a drug with a single compartment and for a drug which distributes to two compartments. For the intravenous plots, the concentration at time = 0 is given.

- Bioavailability is the fraction of drug administered which reaches the systemic circulation.
- Bioavailability (*F*) is calculated from the ratio of the areas under the curve (AUC) of the oral dose to an intravenous dose (Figure 8.1):

$$F = \frac{AUC\ oral}{AUC\ iv}$$

First-pass metabolism
- Some drugs (e.g. propranolol) pass from the gastrointestinal tract to the liver and undergo metabolism before reaching the systemic circulation.
- This reduces bioavailability.
- Some drugs (e.g. glyceryl trinitrate) are given by the buccal route to avoid this.

(Re)distribution

- On entering the body, some drugs are initially dissolved in the plasma but move to other sites (e.g. extracellular space, fat stores). This is distribution.
- Single compartment: the drug remains in the central compartment (plasma).
- Multicompartment: the drug moves out of the plasma to additional sites.

Volume of distribution (V_d)

- V_d of a drug is the apparent or theoretical volume in which a drug is dissolved in the body to give the plasma concentration measured:

$$V_d = \frac{\text{Amount in body}}{\text{Concentration}} = \frac{\text{Dose}}{\text{(Conc.) at } t = 0}$$

- V_d enables a loading dose to be calculated.

Elimination

- Elimination is the removal of the active drug from the body and is made up of hepatic metabolism and renal excretion.

Clearance (CL)

- CL is the volume of plasma cleared of a drug per unit time (ml/min, l/h).

First-order kinetics of elimination

- For most drugs elimination shows first-order kinetics and the plasma concentration undergoes an exponential decay (Figure 8.1).
- The rate of elimination is proportional to the concentration of drug:

$$C_t = C_0 e^{-kt}$$

where C_t = concentration at $t = t$, C_0 = concentration at $t = 0$, k = rate constant (per minute or per hour or per day) and t = time.

Rate constant (k)

- The rate constant (k) is the fraction of drug eliminated per unit time.
- For example, when k is 0.1/day then 10% is eliminated per day.
- This can be applied mathematically as the clearance per unit time and is the fraction of V_d that is cleared per unit time, so:

$$k = \frac{\text{Clearance}}{V_d}$$

or:

$$CL = k \times V_d$$

also:

$$CL = \frac{dose}{AUC}$$

Half-life

The half-life is the time taken for the plasma concentration of a drug to decrease by 50%.

$$t_{1/2} = \frac{\log_e 2}{k} = \frac{0.693}{k}$$

Loading doses

A loading dose is used at the start of some treatments to give a rise in levels to attain therapeutic concentrations. This may be required for drugs with a long half-life (e.g. digoxin) as it takes 5 half-lives to reach steady-state concentrations or drugs where an immediate effect is required (e.g. lidocaine):

Loading dose $=$ target concentration $\times$ V_d

Maintenance doses

At steady state, the maintenance dose equals the amount removed:

Infusion rate $=$ clearance $\times$ C_{ss}

where $C_{ss} =$ concentration at steady state.
- Oral regimen dosing:

$$Dose = \frac{CL \times C_{ss} \times \tau}{F}$$

where τ (tau) is the dosage interval.

Zero-order kinetics
- For some drugs (e.g. phenytoin and ethanol), the enzymes responsible for their elimination become saturated and so the rate of elimination is no longer proportional to the concentration of drug.
- These drugs exhibit zero-order kinetics with the rate of elimination not being proportional to the drug concentration and so small changes in their dosages lead to disproportionate increases in plasma concentrations. The maintenance dose is calculated from the Michaelis–Menten equation:

$$\frac{F \times Dose}{\tau} = \frac{V_{max} \times C_{ss}}{K_m + C_{ss}}$$

where V_{max} and K_m are obtained from population averages.

Drug metabolism

Many drugs undergo metabolism prior to elimination. The process of metabolism usually results in the production of an inactive compound which is more readily excreted. There are exceptions to this:

- Some drugs (known as prodrugs) are activated by metabolism, resulting in more active compounds.
- Some other drug metabolites are pharmacologically active and lead to desired or adverse effects.
- Not all drugs require metabolism prior to excretion.

Drug metabolism is often divided into phase I and phase II. Phase I generally involves oxidation (but may also involve reduction or hydrolysis). Phase II involves conjugation to promote elimination. Phase I and phase II reactions often happen sequentially.

Phase I metabolism

This often involves hepatic oxidation via the cytochrome P450 (CYP450) family. The reactions involve reduced NADP, molecular oxygen and CYP450 isoenzymes.

- CYP450 has many isoenzymes.
- CYP450 enzyme inducers (e.g. carbamazepine, phenobarbital) may increase levels of the enzyme and increase rates of drug metabolism. This leads to drug interactions; for example, carbamazepine may accelerate the metabolism of oral contraceptives, making them ineffective. This type of interaction takes days to develop as the enzymes are induced but may persist for some time after stopping the inducer.
- CYP450 enzyme inhibitors (e.g. erythromycin, cimetidine) may inhibit the metabolism of drugs via the CYP450 systems. The reduced metabolism may lead to higher plasma concentrations of the interacting drugs and promote toxicity. These interactions happen rapidly at the onset of treatment with an inhibitor and reverse once the inhibitor is stopped and has been cleared from the system.
- As there are many CYP450 isoenzymes and several may be involved in the metabolism of drugs, it is difficult to predict which drugs may be affected in this way.

Phase II

This is a transferase reaction and conjugates the drug or metabolite, usually resulting in inactivation. The conjugation usually results in a more polar molecule to facilitate renal or bilary excretion. Reactions include:

- glucuronidation
- methylation
- sulphation
- acetylation
- glutathione conjugates
- amino acid conjugates
- mercapturic acid formation.

Renal elimination

The kidneys are a key site of drug or metabolite elimination. Many drugs are excreted by the weak acid or weak base transporters in the proximal convoluted tubule. These are non-specific transporters which excrete weak acids or bases into the tubular fluid.

- For renally excreted drugs, renal function determines the amount excreted and in renal impairment there is impaired excretion and plasma concentrations rise unless there is dose reduction, e.g. digoxin.
- The weak acid and base transporters are sites of drug interactions, e.g. methotrexate and non-steroidal anti-inflammatory drugs may compete for elimination via weak acid transporters and this may lead to toxicity with methotrexate.
- Some drugs, e.g. thiazide diuretics, require renal excretion to act at the distal convoluted tubule.

KeyEquations

$$t_{1/2} = \frac{\log_e 2}{k}$$

$$CL = V_d \times k$$

$$V_D = \frac{\text{Dose}}{C_{t=0}}$$

Maintenance dose $= CL \times C_{ss}$

$$C_t = C_0 e^{-kt}$$

Self-assessment

In pharmacokinetics, which of the following statements are true or false?

1. A drug with a low volume of distribution is likely to be retained largely in the plasma.
2. Clearance is measured as mass per unit time.
3. Most drugs show first-order kinetics for elimination.
4. If a drug has a rate constant of elimination of 0.05 per day, then 50% of the drug is eliminated per day.
5. If a drug has a rate constant of elimination of 0.05 per hour, then its half-life is about 13.9 h.

chapter 9
Gastric pharmacology

Dyspepsia is the key problem due to acidity:
- gastro-oesophageal reflux disease (GORD), due to reflux of gastric contents into the oesophagus
- peptic ulceration (gastric and duodenal) with erosion, damage, bleeding. Peptic ulceration is largely due to *Helicobacter pylori* infection or induced as an adverse effect of non-steroidal anti-inflammatory drugs (NSAIDs)
- gastritis involves inflammation.

Control of acid secretion

Increase acid secretion:
- histamine via H_2 receptors
- gastrin via cholecystokinin$_2$ receptors
- acetylcholine via M_3 receptors on parietal cells.

Decrease acid secretion:
- prostaglandins (PGE_2 and PGI_2). Also cytoprotective via bicarbonate and mucus release.

Treatment

Antacids
e.g. sodium bicarbonate, aluminium and magnesium hydroxides

Mechanism of action
- As the name implies, they are antiacid and raise pH.
- Sodium bicarbonate is the simplest:
  $HCO_3^- + H^+ \rightarrow CO_2 + H_2O$
- Magnesium hydroxide and aluminium hydroxide are also used:
  $Al(OH)_3 + 3HCl \rightarrow AlCl_3 + 3H_2O$
  $Mg(OH)_2 + 2HCl \rightarrow MgCl_2 + 2H_2O.$

Adverse effects
- Bicarbonate may give rise to wind.
- Magnesium salts lead to diarrhoea.
- Aluminium salts are constipating.

Clinical context
- Antacids provide rapid relief but not cure.

Alginates

- Alginates may be combined with antacids (e.g. Gaviscon).
- The alginic acid, when combined with saliva, forms a viscous foam which floats on the gastric contents, forming a raft which protects the oesophagus during reflux.

Histamine H₂ receptor antagonists

e.g. cimetidine, ranitidine, famotidine

Mechanism of action

- Antagonism of histamine H_2 receptors which are coupled via adenylyl cyclase to increase cyclic adenosine monophosphate (cAMP: see Chapter 3) which activates the proton pump (Figure 9.1).

Figure 9.1 A schematic diagram of a parietal cell showing the control of acid secretion and its modulation via drugs. CCK_2, cholecystokinin$_2$ receptors; ECF, enterochromaffin-like cell; PP, proton pump; PPIs, proton pump inhibitors; PGs, prostaglandins; PGR, prostaglandin receptor; ACh, acetylcholine; NSAIDs, non-steroidal anti-inflammatory drugs; COX, cyclooxygenase; M, muscarinic receptor.

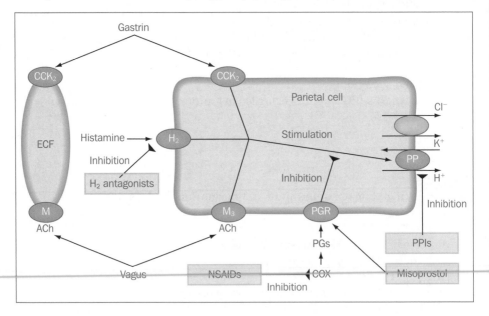

Adverse effects

- Cimetidine inhibits cytochrome P450 and therefore the metabolism of other drugs, resulting in important drug interactions (e.g. oral anticoagulants, phenytoin, carbamazepine, tricyclic antidepressants). Ranitidine does not interact in this way.

Clinical context

- Reduce gastric acid secretion.
- Provide symptomatic relief.

- Best taken at night.
- Promote ulcer healing but there is often relapse on discontinuation.

Proton pump inhibitors (PPIs)
e.g. omeprazole, pantoprazole, lansoprazole

Mechanism of action
- Irreversible inhibition of the proton pump (H^+/K^+-ATPase; see Chapter 4) (Figure 9.1).
- PPIs are activated in an acidic environment which helps selectivity.

Adverse effects
- Inhibit H^+ secretion by >90%, may lead to achlorhydria (absence of acid).
- Increase risk of *Campylobacter* infection (food poisoning) as the stomach acid sterilises food.

Clinical context
- Used for dyspepsia and ulcer healing.
- The most effective antisecretory agents (they inhibit the final common pathway of acid secretion).
- Omeprazole is now available as an over-the-counter medicine.

Prokinetic drugs
- Cause gastric emptying.
- Movement of gastric contents from stomach to duodenum – drugs which do this will be of benefit in GORD.
- Domperidone (dopamine receptor antagonist): increased closure of oesophageal sphincter (good for reflux disease) and opens lower sphincter.
- Metoclopramide (dopamine receptor antagonist): acts locally to increase gastric motility and emptying (combined with analgesics to accelerate absorption).

Helicobacter pylori eradication
- Most peptic ulcers are due to infection with *H. pylori*.
- Eradication is the most effective treatment for long-term cure of ulcers with low relapse rates.
- A variety of combination therapies: 'triple therapy'.
- All involve an antibiotic:
  - two from:
    metronidazole
    amoxicillin
    clarithromycin
  plus
  - PPI and/or H_2 antagonist.

The ulcerogenic effects of NSAIDs (and oral steroids)

- Oral NSAIDS (commonly) and corticosteroids (less commonly) are associated with peptic damage/ulceration.
- NSAIDs inhibit cyclooxygenases (COX; see Chapter 7).
- COX exists as two isoforms:
  - COX-1: physiological, e.g. gastric protection
  - COX-2: pathological, involved in inflammation.
- Most NSAIDs inhibit both and cause gastric damage.
- COX-2-selective inhibitors (celecoxib) were developed to have fewer gastrointestinal side-effects.
- To minimise gastrointestinal damage use a PPI for prophylaxis.
- Give NSAID in combination with misoprostol, a stable prostaglandin E_1 analogue, which acts on prostanoid receptors to inhibit gastric H^+ secretion

KeyPoints

- Most ulcers are due to *H. pylori* infection.
- NSAID-induced gastric damage is one of the most important adverse drug reactions.
- Antacids provide rapid relief in simple indigestion.
- PPIs are the most effective agents.
- *H. pylori*-induced ulceration may be cured by triple therapy (of two antibiotics and a PPI).

(Figure 9.1).

Self-assessment

1. Which of the following statements are true or false regarding peptic ulceration?
a. Infection with *H. pylori* is the most common cause.
b. Triple therapy is the combination of an antacid, an H_2 receptor antagonist and a proton pump inhibitor.
c. NSAIDs cause ulceration via COX-2 inhibition.
d. Misoprostol makes NSAID-induced ulceration worse.

2. Which of the following may reduce gastric acid secretion?
a. histamine H_1 receptor antagonists
b. agents that increase cAMP
c. gastrin
d. PPIs

chapter 10
Lower gastrointestinal pharmacology

Drugs which affect the lower gastrointestinal tract are used to manage diarrhoea, constipation, irritable-bowel syndrome and inflammatory bowel disease.

Diarrhoea

- This is the passing of frequent (more than three per day), watery or soft stools and is a common, debilitating condition that can be life-threatening in vulnerable patients due to dehydration.
- Acute diarrhoea is usually due to either a bacterial or viral infection:
  - Rotavirus: these damage small-bowel villi.
  - Invasive bacteria: these damage epithelium. Some bacteria (e.g. *Campylobacter*) release cytotoxins which damage the muscosa.
- Adhesive enterotoxigenic bacteria (such as cholera) release toxins, which adhere to brush border and permanently activate adenylyl cyclase, increasing cyclic adenosine monophosphate (cAMP), which leads to Cl^- and Na^+ secretion followed by water.
- Diarrhoea may be secondary to drugs:
  - Antibiotics may alter the natural intestinal flora, allowing the outgrowth of pathogenic bacteria, leading to an infection with diarrhoea. This commonly complicates the use of broad-spectrum antibiotics.
  - Orlistat (used in obesity; see Chapter 16) is a pancreatic lipase inhibitor and so prevents the breakdown of fat, leading to oily diarrhoea (steatorrhoea).
  - Misoprostol (used in gastroprotection; see Chapter 9) can lead to diarrhoea.
  - Proton pump inhibitors reduce gastric acid secretion and, as acid sterilises the gastric contents, its absence can promote infections.

Oral rehydration therapy
- The most effective treatment: it involves a solution of electrolytes to replace those lost in diarrhoea.
- The glucose allows epithelial transport of sodium via a symporter and this is followed by water, leading to rehydration (Figure 10.1).

Antimotility agents (opioids)
e.g. codeine and loperamide

Figure 10.1 A gut epithelial cell demonstrating the effects of oral rehydration therapy via glucose promoting the uptake of sodium, which is followed by water, leading to rehydration.

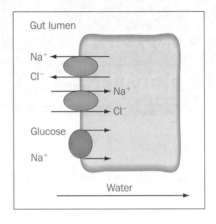

Mechanism of action

- Antimotility agents reduce tone and peristaltic movements of gastrointestinal muscle by presynaptic inhibition (via μ-opioid receptors; Figure 10.2).

Figure 10.2 Schematic diagram of a parasympathetic nerve ending showing presynaptic inhibition of acetylcholine (ACh) release due to negative coupling of μ-opioid receptors to adenylyl cyclase (AC), and the activation of potassium conductance and hyperpolarisation.

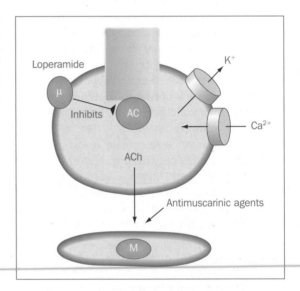

- Presynaptic inhibition is via an increased potassium conductance (hyperpolarisation), which reduces calcium influx and this reduces the release of acetylcholine, which reduces motility and increases transit time and promotes reabsorption of water.

Clinical context

- These agents provide symptomatic relief only and do not reduce the length of a bout of diarrhoea.
- Loperamide does not penetrate the blood–brain barrier and has an efficient enterohepatic cycling, so is retained largely in the gut. Hence loperamide is devoid of central opioid effects (see Chapter 25).

- All opioids are constipating via this mechanism – a key side-effect of opioid treatment.

Antimotility agents: antimuscarinic agents
e.g. dicycloverine
- These block the postjunctional muscarininc receptors on the smooth muscle, leading to reduced motility.
- Tricyclic antidepressants (TCAs) are also constipating as a side-effect through antagonism of muscarinic receptors.

Constipation

- Constipation is altered bowel habits with fewer than three motions a week.
- The cause may be a diet lacking in roughage and the condition may often be managed by a balanced diet.
- The cause may be drug-induced:
  - opioids (see above)
  - TCAs (see above)
  - antimuscarinic drugs (see above)
  - diuretics (due to dehydration).

Laxatives
- Osmotic laxatives include lactulose (a disaccharide of galactose and fructose) which enters the colon unchanged and is converted by bacteria to lactic acid and acetic acid and raises fluid volume osmotically.
- Magnesium salts have an osmotic effect and may release cholecystokinin to increase gastrointestinal motility.
- Bulking agents (e.g. ispaghula, methylcellulose) increase the bulk of faecal matter and so increase motility.
- Stimulant laxatives (e.g. senna extracts) enter the colon and are metabolised to derivatives, which stimulate gastrointestinal activity.

Irritable-bowel syndrome

This is a common, long-standing disorder and may involve pain and bloating, which are relieved by defecation. There may be episodes of diarrhoea and/or constipation.

Treatment may involve:
- lactulose or loperamide for symptoms
- antispasmodic agents such as antimuscarinics, which inhibit parasympathetic activity, or mebeverine, which is a direct relaxant of gastrointestinal smooth muscle
- amitriptyline (a TCA) is widely used in low doses and provides some pain relief, has antimuscarinic effects and may alter the sensitivity of sensory nerves.

Inflammatory bowel disease

This includes Crohn's disease and ulcerative colitis, which are characterised by chronic inflammation with pain and bloody diarrhoea. These conditions are managed via anti-inflammatories and immunosuppressants.

5-Aminosalicylates
e.g. sulphasalazine, mesalazine
- These agents release 5-aminosalicylate (5-ASA).
- 5-ASA inhibits leukotriene and prostanoid formation, scavenges free radicals and decreases neutrophil chemotaxis.

Corticosteroids (see Chapter 33)
- Anti-inflammatory, immunosuppressive actions.
- Budesonide is used as it is poorly absorbed and so has far fewer systemic side-effects.

Immunosuppressants
- Azathioprine, ciclosporin and methotrexate are used.
- Infliximab is a monoclonal antibody directed against tumour necrosis factor-α and is used in severe Crohn's disease.

Key Points

- Diarrhoea is best managed by oral rehydration therapy.
- Broad-spectrum antibiotics often cause diarrhoea as a side-effect.
- Opioids (such as loperamide) cause presynaptic inhibition to reduce gastrointestinal motility. They provide symptomatic relief but do not shorten a bout of diarrhoea.
- Opioids are constipating via the above mechanism.
- Drugs with antimuscarinic actions are constipating.
- Laxatives are osmotic, bulk or stimulating.
- Inflammatory bowel disease is managed via anti-inflammatories and immunosuppressants.

Self-assessment

1. **Which of the following are likely to cause diarrhoea?**
a. broad-spectrum antibiotics
b. opioid agonists
c. muscarinic receptor antagonists
d. orlistat

2. **Which of the following are likely to cause constipation?**
a. broad-spectrum antibiotics
b. opioid agonists
c. muscarinic receptor antagonists
d. orlistat

chapter 11
Antiemetics

A range of stimuli (e.g. motion) and toxins (alcohol, drugs, e.g. anticancer drugs, opioids bacterial toxins) cause nausea, leading to vomiting. There are several mechanisms of nausea, including local irritation of the stomach involving visceral afferent fibres, the central effects of toxins on the chemoreceptor trigger zone (CTZ) and the conflict between visual and balance information, which is thought to occur in motion sickness. The vomiting pathway is under common, central control leading to a highly co-ordinated physiological response. Vomiting is under the control of the vomiting centre, which receives a direct input from visceral afferent nerves and is also regulated by the CTZ. The CTZ is, in turn, sensitive to circulating drugs and toxins, and receives input from the vestibular nuclei, linked to the labyrinth of the inner ear.

Histamine H_1 receptor antagonists

e.g. cinnarizine, cyclizine, promethazine
- Histamine H_1 receptor antagonism and antimuscarinic effects lead to antiemetic effects.
- They act on the vestibular nuclei.
- They are effective in motion sickness.

Antimuscarinic agents

e.g. hyoscine
- Antimuscarinic agencts act in both the vomiting centre and the vestibular apparatus.
- They are highly effective in motion sickness.
- Substantial antimuscarinic side-effects limit their usefulness.

Histamine analogues

e.g. betahistine
- Histamine H_1 receptor partial agonist and H_3 receptor antagonist may increase blood flow to the inner ear and/or decrease endolymph pressure.
- Used in vertigo and Ménière's disease.

Dopamine receptor antagonists

e.g. domperidone, metoclopramide, phenothiazines such as prochlorperazine

- Dopamine receptor antagonists block D_2 dopamine receptors in the CTZ.
- They may have unwanted central nervous system (CNS) effects (less so with domperidone), which may include extrapyramidal effects and drug-induced parkinsonism.
- Metoclopramide is also a $5HT_3$-receptor antagonist and a $5HT_4$ receptor agonist.
- The prokinetic effects of domperidone and metoclopramide may increase gastric emptying, and are useful for feelings of fullness and nausea.
- They are effective against anticancer drug-induced emesis.
- Domperidone prevents nausea due to dopamine receptor agonists and levodopa used in Parkinson's disease.

5-hydroxytryptamine (5HT) receptor antagonists

e.g. ondansetron (also metoclopramide)

- These block 5HT, acting at $5HT_3$ receptors in the gut and CTZ.
- They are particularly effective against anticancer drugs, which may cause the release of 5HT in the gastrointestinal tract.
- They are effective in postoperative nausea and vomiting.

Other agents

These include corticosteroids (e.g. dexamethasone) and a cannabinoid receptor agonist (nabilone). In both cases the mechanism of action is unclear.

KeyPoints

- There is a range of agents with different sites of action. The site of action determines the clinical effectiveness.
- Targets include muscarinic, histamine H_1, dopamine D_2 and $5\text{-}HT_3$ receptors.

Self-assessment

Which of the following classes of drugs are associated with antiemetic effects?
1. histamine H_2 receptor antagonists
2. $5HT_2$ agonists
3. dopamine receptor agonists
4. muscarinic receptor antagonists
5. dopamine D_2 receptor antagonists
6. opioids

chapter 12
Antiarrhythmics

Arrhythmias are common disorders of cardiac excitation, which may be benign but may also be fatal (e.g. ventricular fibrillation following a heart attack). Antiarrhythmic drugs may be used to control or correct cardiac rhythm. The problems and types of arrhythmia are summarised below.

Too slow a heart rate

- This can occur in heart block, where there is impaired conduction at the atrioventricular node (AVN). Block may be complete or partial.
- It can be drug-induced (e.g. digoxin).

Too short a time for filling

- This can occur in fast atrial fibrillation: the sinoatrial node (SAN) is no longer the principal pacemaker and there are multiple sites of abnormal electrical activity, resulting in atrial fibrillation and some of the impulses are conducted to the ventricles increasing heart rate. Anticoagulation is required due to the risk of emboli forming, which can pass to the cerebral circulation leading to a stroke.
- Multiple supraventricular ectopics: these are abnormal impulses conducted from the atria to ventricles (as in atrial flutter), resulting in increased heart rate (supraventricular tachycardia).
- Accessory pathways: anatomical pathways not at the AVN which conduct impulses from the atria to ventricles. These pathways are faster and have shorter refractory periods than the AVN. These are a form of re-entrant arrhythmias, where impulses may recirculate and lead to abnormal beats. Other forms of re-entrant arrhythmias involve an impulse bypassing a less excitable area and then re-exciting that area retrogradely with a circus of electrical activity.
- Ventricular ectopic beats: abnormal impulses generated in the ventricles from ectopic pacemakers, leading to palpitations.

Risk of progression to fatal arrhythmias

- Torsades de pointes: QRS complexes on the electrocardiogram of varying amplitudes may lead to ventricular fibrillation.
- Ventricular fibrillation: this is totally unco-ordinated cardiac excitation and contraction, leading to no concerted cardiac output.

The cardiac action potential

- This varies from region to region, with SAN tissue having the highest intrinsic rate.
- Ventricular tissue has a prolonged plateau of depolarisation (open voltage-operated calcium channels) to facilitate contraction in systole.
- Understanding the currents in the action potential (Figure 12.1) is essential to appreciate the mechanism of antiarrhythmic drugs.

Figure 12.1 Idealised action potentials in (a) a sinoatrial node pacemaker cell and (b) a ventricular cell.

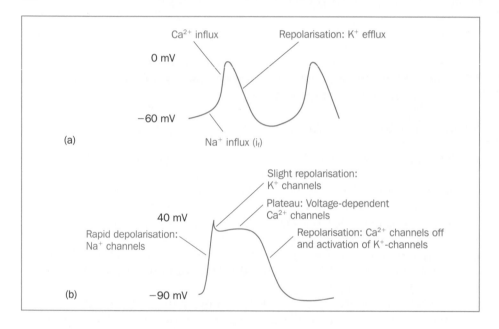

Autonomic control of the heart

- Sympathetic: noradrenaline (and circulating adrenaline) act at β_1-adrenoceptors (coupled to increased cyclic adenosine monophosphate (cAMP); see Chapter 3) to cause increases in force (positive inotropic) and rate (positive chronotropic) of contraction.
- Parasympathetic: acetylcholine from the vagus acts on M_2 muscarinic receptors (negatively coupled to cAMP but positively to an increase in K^+ conductance; see Chapter 3) to slow the pacemaker at the SAN and slow AV conduction. This slows the heart rate (negative chronotropic).

Antiarrhythmic drugs

Antiarrhythmic drugs are categorised into four classes:

Class I

- Local anaesthetics which cause use-dependent blockade of fast Na^+ channels.
- Reduce rate of rise of action potential, decrease rate of conduction and prolong refractory period:
  - class Ia: procainamide, quinidine, disopyramide: kinetics intermediate between Ib and Ic
  - class Ib: lidocaine: fast dissociation
  - class Ic: flecainide: slow dissociation.
- Used in ventricular tachycardia.

Class II

e.g. atenolol, propranolol

- β-adrenoceptor antagonists and so block effects of sympathetic nervous system. Slows pacemaker.
- Reduces proarrhythmic effects of catecholamines.
- May also possess some class I activity.
- Improves survival post myocardial infarction.

Class III

e.g. amiodarone

- Block K^+-channels.
- Prolong action potential and so refractory period.
- Sotalol is a β-blocker which also has class III activity.
- Used in supraventricular and ventricular tachycardia.

Class IV

e.g. verapamil, diltiazem

- Block L-type voltage-dependent Ca^{2+}-channels associated with cardiac action potential.
- Slow conduction at the AVN and are known as rate-limiting calcium channel blockers.
- Dihydropyridine calcium channel antagonists do not act on the heart and are not antiarrhythmic.
- Reduce heart rate and force of contraction.
- Useful in supraventricular tachycardia.

In addition:

Digoxin

- Inhibits $3Na^+/2K^+$ ATPase (sodium pump) (see Chapter 4).
- Is a direct AVN block and also causes vagal activation which induces a degree of heart block. This controls the ventricular rate and so is useful in atrial fibrillation.

Adenosine

- Activates A_1 adenosine receptors to activate K^+ channels (acetylcholine-sensitive M-current) and cause hyperpolarisation of the AVN.

- Induces heart/conduction block.
- Used to terminate supraventricular tachycardia.

Magnesium chloride
- Mechanism poorly understood.
- Causes calcium channel blockade.

KeyPoints _____

- Class I: Na^+-channel inhibitors.
- Class II: β-blockers.
- Class III: K^+-channel inhibitors.
- Class IV: Ca^{2+}-channel inhibitors.
- Digoxin is an Na-pump inhibitor used in atrial fibrillation.

Self-assessment

1. **Concerning antiarrhythmic drugs, which of the following are true or false?**
a. Class I agents are local anaesthetics
b. Class I agents show use dependence
c. Class II agents (β-blockers) improve survival post myocardial infarction
d. Digoxin improves AVN conduction
e. Digoxin reduces calcium entry into cells

2. **Which of the following will reduce heart rate?**
a. Calcium channel antagonists (such as verapamil)
b. Dihydropyridine calcium channel antagonists (such as nifedipine)
c. Antimuscarinic agents
d. Digoxin
e. β-adrenoceptor agonists

chapter 13
Cardiovascular drugs

Cardiovascular drugs act on the heart or blood vessels to control the cardiovascular system. They are used to treat a variety of conditions from hypertension to heart failure.

- Hypertension: an increase in blood pressure (typically systolic blood pressure > 140 mmHg and diastolic blood pressure > 90 mmHg but decisions to treat are based on overall cardiovascular risk). Hypertension is associated with causing strokes, ischaemic heart disease, chronic heart failure (CHF) and renal damage and therapy aims to reduce these risks.
- Ischaemic heart disease includes angina (where coronary blood flow is impaired) and myocardial infarction.
- CHF is impaired cardiac function where the pump activity of the heart is insufficient for the body's demands.

Angiotensin-converting enzyme inhibitors (ACEIs)

e.g. enalapril, lisinopril, ramipril

Mechanism of action (Figure 13.1)
- ACEIs inhibit the conversion of angiotensin I to angiotensin II by inhibiting angiotensin-converting enzyme (ACE), which is predominantly in the lungs.
- Angiotensin II is a vasoconstrictor (directly, and indirectly via enhancing sympathetic activity).
- Angiotensin II increases the release of aldosterone (sodium/fluid-retaining and potassium-losing hormone).

Figure 13.1 Flow diagram of the renin–angiotensin–aldosterone pathway and the actions of angiotensin-converting enzyme (ACE) inhibitors to reduce the conversion of angiotensin (AI) to angiotensin II (AII).

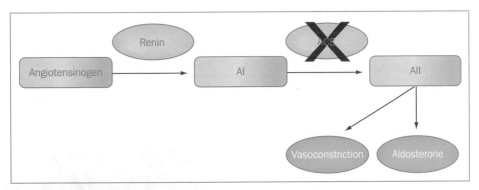

- ACE is also involved in the breakdown of bradykinin (an endogenous vasodilator) and so ACEIs will increase bradykinin levels.
- ACEIs reduce angiotensin II-induced vasoconstriction and indirectly aldosterone-induced sodium/fluid retention and so lower blood pressure and fluid overload.

Adverse effects

- A dry cough (10% of patients) may be present due to increased bradykinin levels. This may result in the patient changing to an angiotensin AT_1 receptor antagonist (see below).
- Renal damage may occur, especially in patients with renovascular disease, where angiotensin II is elevated to maintain renal blood flow and an ACEI will lead to reduced renal flow and severe hypotension.
- First-dose hypotension: this is a large drop in blood pressure at the start of therapy – patients are advised to take the first dose when retiring to bed.
- Hyperkalaemia (increased plasma K^+), due to inhibition of aldosterone (K^+-losing hormone). This is especially a problem when used with potassium-sparing diuretics (see Chapter 14) or with potassium chloride as a salt substitute.

Clinical context

- Hypertension: first choice for hypertension in patients under 55 years of age.
- Diabetic nephropathy: reduce renal damage in diabetes.
- CHF: first-choice drug for reducing symptoms and mortality. ACEIs may reverse or prevent the adverse effects of angiotensin II in CHF (which forms part of adverse neurohormonal adaptation).
- Ischaemic heart disease and post myocardial infarction: routinely used to reduce mortality.

Angiotensin (AT_1) receptor antagonists

'sartans', e.g. losartan

Mechanism of action (Figure 13.2)

Figure 13.2 Flow diagram of the renin–agniotensin–aldosterone pathway and the actions of an angiotensin II AT_1 receptor antagonist to oppose the actions of angiotensin II (AII). AI, angiotensin I; ACE, antiotensin-converting enzyme.

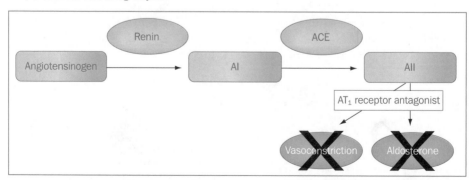

- Competitive antagonism of the actions of angiotensin II at the AT_1 receptor. Angiotensin II acts at AT_1 (vasoconstriction and aldosterone releases) and AT_2 receptors (roles are uncertain but may be important in the fetus).
- They have the same consequences as ACEIs but do not affect bradykinin levels.

Adverse effects
- Same as ACEIs but do not cause a cough.

Clinical context
- Used when ACEIs are not tolerated due to cough.
- Sometimes used with ACEIs for dual blockade, but this increases the risk of side-effects.

Beta-blockers

e.g. atenolol

Mechanism of action
- Competitive antagonists of β_1- and β_2-adrenoceptors and so oppose the actions of noradrenaline from sympathetic nerves and circulating adrenaline.
- β-adrenoceptors: G-protein-coupled receptors which activate adenylyl cyclase and increase cyclic adenosine monophosphate (cAMP; see Chapter 3).
  - β_1-adrenoceptors: heart, coupled to increases in force of contraction (positive inotropic) and heart rate (positive chronotropic) (see Chapter 12).
  - β_2-adrenoceptors: lungs, coupled to bronchodilatation (see Chapter 17), and on blood vessels, coupled to vasodilatation.
- β-blockers act at β_1- and β_2-adrenoceptors to varying degrees. Cardioselective ones (e.g. atenolol) are selective for β_1-adrenoceptors but may have some action at β_2-adrenoceptors. Older agents (e.g. propranolol) are non-selective.
- Hypertension: the mechanism is uncertain but may decrease cardiac output (blockade of cardiac β_1-adrenoceptors), may reduce renin release (blockade of β-adrenoceptors on renal juxtaglomerular cells) and may have central actions.
- Angina: reduce heart rate and so cardiac work. The reduction in heart rate increases the time for diastole, during which coronary flow occurs, and so improves coronary blood flow.

Adverse effects
- Blockade of bronchial β_2-adrenoceptors can cause bronchoconstriction, even with cardioselective agents, and so β-blockers are avoided in patients with asthma.
- Cold peripheries due to blockade of vasodilator β_2-adrenoceptors.
- Impotence.

Clinical context

- Angina: reduced cardiac work and improved coronary blood flow mean that β-blockers are first-choice drugs for prevention.
- Post myocardial infarction: used after a heart attack to reduce mortality.
- Certain cardioselective agents (metoprolol, bisoprolol, carvedilol) are now used in CHF as they oppose the adverse effects of noradrenaline in neurohormonal adaptation and are proven to reduce mortality. They are used with caution, starting at a low dose and titrating upwards as β-blockers initially reduce cardiac output and cause a worsening of CHF at the start of treatment.
- Hypertension: no longer used as first-choice drugs as they are less effective at reducing stroke, heart attack, heart failure and diabetes compared to ACEIs, diuretics and calcium channel blockers.
- Antiarrhythmic: reduce sympathetic drive to heart.
- Anxiety: block the sympathetic component of anxiety.
- Hyperthyroidism: reduce initial symptoms due to increased sympathetic activity.
- Migraine: for prevention.
- Glaucoma: as topical agents which reduce pressure in the eye.

Diuretics

Although these act on the kidney, they are widely used in cardiovascular disease to reduce extracellular volume and/or oedema (see Chapter 14).

Calcium channel inhibitors

1. Dihydropyridines, e.g. amlodipine, nifedipine
2. Rate-limiting, e.g. verapamil.

Mechanism of action (Figure 13.3)

Figure 13.3 Mechanisms of action of vasodilators (nitrates, calcium channel inhibitors and a K_{ATP} channel activator, nicorandil) on vascular smooth muscle. cGMP, cyclic guanosine monophosphate; sGC, soluble guanylyl cyclase.

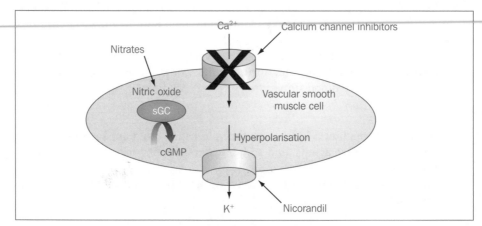

- Calcium channel inhibitors inhibit calcium channels and so reduce calcium entry to contractile smooth muscle and cardiac muscle.
- Dihydropyridines are selective for calcium channels on vascular smooth muscle and so cause vasodilatation.
- Rate-limiting agents have greater activity on cardiac muscle and so reduce the force of cardiac contraction and heart rate (see Chapter 12).

Adverse effects
- Dihydropyridines: arteriolar vasodilatation may lead to increases in fluid leaving the circulation, resulting in ankle oedema.
- Verapamil: inhibition of calcium channels in gastrointestinal smooth muscle can lead to constipation.

Clinical context
- Hypertension: first-choice drugs for patients over 55 years. Act via vasodilatation and, in the case of the rate-limiting agents, also via reducing cardiac output.
- Angina: due to vasodilatation which reduces cardiac work and coronary vasodilatation which will increase coronary blood flow. Rate-limiting agents also reduce heart rate, reducing cardiac work and increasing time for diastole (and so increasing coronary flow).
- Antiarrhythmic: rate-limiting agents acting via inhibition of cardiac calcium channels.

Nitrates

e.g. glyceryl trinitrate, isosorbide mononitrate

Mechanism of action (Figure 13.3)
- Release nitric oxide which acts on soluble guanylyl cyclase to increase cyclic guanosine monophosphate (cGMP) to cause vasodilatation.
- Vasodilatation is predominantly venous.
- Angina: increased venodilatation reduces venous return (return of blood to the heart) and so reduces cardiac work. May also cause coronary vasodilatation.

Adverse effects
- Vasodilatation may lead to a throbbing headache which should respond to paracetamol.
- Nitrate tolerance: continued exposure to nitrates (usually oral agents such as mononitrates) can result in them becoming less effective. A nitrate-free period (e.g. overnight) can reduce the risk of tolerance.

Clinical context
- Glyceryl trinitrate for sublingual administration (e.g. a spray) causes rapid relief of angina.
- Oral nitrates (e.g. isosorbide mononitrate) may be used for regular prevention in angina.

Potassium channel activators

e.g. nicorandil

Mechanism of action (Figure 13.3)
- Potassium channel activators activate adenosine triphosphate (ATP)-sensitive potassium (K_{ATP}) channels on vascular smooth muscle (see Chapter 4).
- The opening of these K_{ATP} channels causes K^+ to leave the smooth muscle, resulting in hyperpolarisation, which causes the cells to become less excitable, and this results in vasorelaxation.

Adverse effects
- The vasodilatation can result in a reflex increase in heart rate.

Clinical context
- Nicorandil is used in angina for its vasodilator actions.

Alpha-blockers

e.g. prazosin

Mechanism of action
- Competitive antagonists of α_1-adrenoceptors and so block sympathetic-mediated vasoconstriction, leading to vasodilatation.

Adverse effects
- Numerous, due to blockade of the sympathetic nervous system, and this limits their tolerability and usage.
- Postural or orthostatic hypotension, due to blockade of sympathetic nervous system, and so the patient is unable to maintain blood pressure when getting up.
- Reflex tachycardia: hypotensive action provokes a reflex increase in heart rate.

Clinical context
- Hypertension: α-blockers are added to therapy when other agents have failed to control blood pressure.
- Prostatic hypertrophy: they are used to reduce symptoms of poor urinary outflow and urgency when the prostate is enlarged, which is common in males over the age of 50 years.

Centrally acting antihypertensive

e.g. α-methyldopa, moxonidine, clonidine

Mechanisms of action

- Thought to decrease sympathetic drive and/or increase vagal output from central cardiovascular control centres.
- α-methyldopa: a false substrate resulting in an analogue of noradrenaline acting at central α_2-adrenoceptors.
- Moxonidine: an imidazoline which activates central imidazoline receptors.
- Clonidine: an α_2-adrenoceptor agonist which acts centrally to decrease sympathetic output.

Clinical context

- Hypertension: these agents are not widely used due to widespread side-effects and no advantages over other antihypertensive agents.
- Hypertension in pregnancy: α-methyldopa is sometimes used as it appears safe in pregnancy.

Cardiac glycosides

Digoxin

- Inhibition of the sodium pump ($3Na^+/2K^+$ ATPase).
- Inhibition of sodium pump in cardiac cells leads to Na^+ accumulation in the cells (Figure 13.4). This increases intracellular Na^+ and so reduces the rate of Ca^{2+} efflux which is driven via a Na^+/Ca^{2+} exchanger. The reduced Ca^{2+} efflux leads to increased intracellular Ca^{2+}, leading to an increase in the force of contraction (positive inotrope).
- Acts on the atrioventricular node (AVN) to cause a degree of conduction block which is of benefit in atrial fibrillation.
- Increases vagal activity, which slows the heart and induces a degree of AVN block.

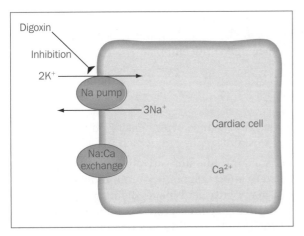

Figure 13.4 Actions of digoxin on the sodium pump of a cardiac cell, leading to increased intracellular calcium.

Clinical context

- Digoxin has a narrow therapeutic window and so is predisposed towards toxicity (nausea, anorexia, visual disturbances, cardiac arrhythmias).
- It used to be widely used in CHF for its positive inotropic actions but is now reserved for CHF with atrial fibrillation or when CHF patients are refractory to other treatments.
- The actions of digoxin are enhanced in hypokalaemia when the sodium pump is less active due to reduced levels of potassium.
- Digoxin is largely renally excreted and renal function is measured during treatment to determine the appropriate dose.

HMG CoA reductase inhibitors (statins)

e.g. simvastatin, pravastatin

Mechanism of action

The statins inhibit the hepatic enzyme, hydroxyl-methylglutaryl coenzyme A reductase (HMG CoA reductase), which catalyses the first committed step of cholesterol synthesis in the liver. This leads to a reduction in cholesterol synthesis.

Adverse effects

Very occasionally they may cause muscle damage. In severe cases the muscle may break down, releasing myoglobin, which can lead to renal damage.

Clinical context

- These are cholesterol-lowering drugs given to patients with a high cardiovascular risk (previous heart attack, ischaemic heart disease, hypertension, diabetes) or abnormally high cholesterol levels to reduce overall risk.
- Simvastatin is now an over-the-counter medicine.
- Most statins are given at night when cholesterol synthesis is greatest.
- They have limited effects in hypertriglyceridaemia.

Fibrates

e.g. bezafibrate, fenofibrate

Mechanism of action

- Fibrates are activators of peroxisome proliferator-activated receptor alpha (PPAR-α; see Chapter 2) and lead to alterations in lipoprotein metabolism.
- This results in the induction of many fatty acid-metabolising enzymes, including peripheral lipoprotein lipases, which promote the breakdown of very-low-density lipoprotein (VLDL: with small reductions in low-density lipoprotein (LDL) and increases in high-density lipoprotein (HDL)) and also lead to reductions in triglycerides.

Adverse effects

Very occasionally they may cause muscle damage and the risk is increased when used with statins.

Clinical context

- Used in hypertriglyceridaemia.

KeyPoints

- Cardiovascular drugs have a range of clinical uses (from hypertension to heart failure).
- Key targets involve interfering with the sympathetic nervous system (e.g. blockade of adreno-ceptors), inhibiting the renin–angiotensin–aldosterone system (ACEIs) and reducing excitability of vascular smooth muscle or cardiac muscle (calcium channel inhibitors).
- Hypertension: ACEIs, calcium channel inhibitors and thiazide diuretics are first-line agents.
- Ischaemic heart disease: β-blockers are first-line and calcium channel inhibitors are second-line drugs. Glyceryl trinitrate spray is used to relieve attacks.
- CHF: ACEI and diuretics play major roles. Certain β-blockers have been shown to improve outcome.
- Digoxin is used in CHF with atrial fibrillation or in refractory CHF.
- Statins are effective at reducing cardiovascular risk, even in patients with 'normal' cholesterol levels.

Self-assessment

1. **Which one of the following is a reason to avoid using an ACEI?**
a. heart failure
b. hypokalaemia (low plasma potassium)
c. renovascular disease
d. asthma

2. **Which one of the following is a reason to avoid using a β-blocker?**
a. hypertension
b. hypokalaemia (low plasma potassium)
c. renovascular disease
d. asthma

3. **Which one of the following is thought to contribute towards the antianginal effects of β-blockers?**
a. reduced release of noradrenaline
b. local anaesthetic effects on sensory nerves
c. reduction in the heart rate with prolongation of diastolic time
d. direct coronary vasodilatation

4. **Which one of the following is unlikely to occur with verapamil?**
a. increase in heart rate
b. reduced force of cardiac contraction

   c. fall in blood pressure

   d. constipation

5. Which of the following is inhibited by digoxin?

   a. ATP-sensitive potassium channels

   b. proton pump

   c. sodium pump

   d. calcium channels

chapter 14
Renal and urinary pharmacology

Diuretics

These are drugs which generally increase Na^+ excretion (natriuresis) in the kidney and the excreted Na^+ is followed osmotically by water. They are used to decrease extracellular/plasma volume and so reduce oedema. They are important cardiovascular drugs used in the treatment of hypertension and chronic heart failure.

Osmotic diuretics
e.g. mannitol
- These are pharmacologically inert and freely filtered at Bowman's capsule.
- They increase osmolality of tubular fluid in proximal convoluted tubule and loop of Henle and so reduce passive reabsorption of H_2O.
- They are used in cerebral oedema as the increased osmolality removes fluid from the brain.

Loop diuretics
e.g. furosemide (frusemide), bumetanide
- These are 'high-ceiling' diuretics which have a very powerful diuretic effect and can cause 15–25% of filtered Na^+ to be excreted.
- They block $Na^+/2Cl^-/K^+$ symporter of the thick ascending limb of the loop of Henle (Figure 14.1).
- They reduce the ability of the loop of Henle to concentrate urine by preventing creation of a hypertonic interstitium in the medulla.

Adverse effects
- Loop diuretics increase Na^+ delivery to distal convoluted tubule (DCT) which promotes K^+ loss (leading to hypokalaemia).
- They decrease Na^+ entry into macula densa which promotes renin release and increases angiotensin II activity.
- Loss of transepithelial potential reduces absorption of divalent cations and causes the loss of Ca^{2+} and Mg^{2+}.
- Postural hypotension (this may lead to falls) may arise due to volume depletion.

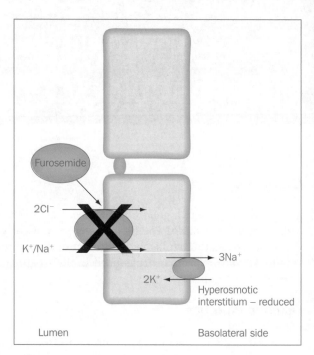

Figure 14.1 Mechanism of action of a loop diuretic.

Clinical context

- Loop diuretics are used in chronic heart failure: they reduce pulmonary oedema secondary to left ventricular failure and peripheral oedema.
- They are venodilators and have a rapid effect in acute left ventricular failure.
- They are used in renal failure to improve diuresis.

Thiazides

e.g. bendroflumethiazide

- Thiazides are moderately powerful diuretics which act on the DCT.
- They inhibit active Na^+ reabsorption and accompanying Cl^-. This increases solute in tubular fluid and so decreases the gradient for water reabsorption.

Adverse effects

- Cause K^+ loss (hypokalaemia).
- Cause metabolic disturbances, leading to impaired glucose control which may lead to diabetes.
- Postural hypotension due to volume depletion. This may lead to falls.

Clinical context

- First-line drugs in hypertension (for patients > 55 years).
- Also used in mild to moderate heart failure.
- Thiazides are renally excreted prior to acting on DCT and so are ineffective in moderate renal impairment.

Hypokalaemia and diuretics (Figure 14.2)

- Loop diuretics and thiazide cause K^+ loss which leads to hypokalaemia, a major clinical problem:
  - more negative membrane potential (hyperpolarisation)
  - predisposes to cardiac arrhythmias
  - potentiates the action of digoxin.
- Diuretics activate the renin–angiotensin–aldosterone system via:
  - decreased Na^+ in extracellular fluid
  - loops block NaCl entry into macula densa
  - volume depletion.
- Activation of the renin–angiotensin–aldosterone system stimulates the release of aldosterone.
- Aldosterone induces the expression of Na^+ channels in the apical (luminal) membranes and Na^+ pumps (aldosterone-induced proteins) in the basolateral membranes of DCT cells and the collecting duct. It is Na^+ retaining at the expense of K^+.

Figure 14.2 (a) The actions of aldosterone which lead to aldosterone-induced proteins (AIPs); (b) the actions of AIPs (sodium channels and sodium pumps which promote sodium retention and potassium loss in distal convoluted tubule cells). AII, angiotensin II; N, nucleus.

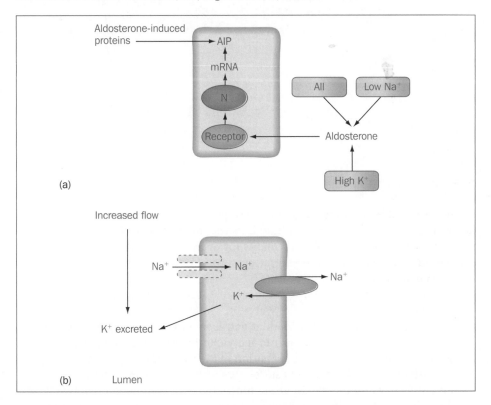

Potassium-sparing diuretics

These are weak diuretics that are used in combination with loop diuretics or thiazides to reduce the risk of hypokalaemia. They include:
- Na^+ channel blockers
- aldosterone (mineralocorticoid) receptor antagonists.

Angiotensin-converting enzyme (ACE) inhibitors (see Chapter 13) cause hyperkalaemia and so may negate the effects of K-losing diuretics.

Aldosterone (mineralocorticoid) receptor antagonists

e.g. spironolactone
- Antagonise mineralocorticoid (MR) (or aldosterone) receptors.
- Prevent insertion of Na^+ pumps and channels.

Sodium channel blockers

e.g. amiloride and triamterene
- Block luminal Na^+ channels in DCT and collecting duct (Figure 14.3).
- Na^+ is no longer retained at expense of K^+.

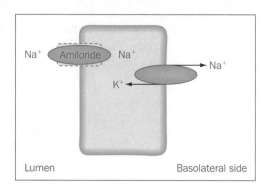

Figure 14.3 The blockade of an apical sodium channel in a distal convoluted tubule cell, reducing potassium loss.

Bladder pharmacology

Overactive bladder involves urgency, sometimes with incontinence and nocturia. It is a widespread condition, affecting more than 10% of adults; incidence increases with age. Treatments for overactive bladder include dietary changes (avoidance of caffeine and reduced fluid intake) as well as physical training such as pelvic floor exercises.
- The mainstay of drug therapy is the use of antimuscarinic drugs, such as darifenacin, tolterodine and oxybutynin. These act to reduce the parasympathetic tone in the bladder detrusor smooth muscle. Whilst all these agents have modest M_3 muscarinic acetylcholine receptor antagonist selectivity, the widespread distribution of M_3 receptors and the lack of selectivity means that patients suffer other effects of the medication, including dry mouth, constipation, blurred vision, mental confusion and drowsiness. These effects may be relatively minor or transient, in comparison with the discomfort or psychological distress of the untreated condition.

- Duloxetine is a serotonin and noradrenaline reuptake inhibitor (SNRI) used for the treatment of stress incontinence, that is, where physical strain, such as sneezing, gives rise to incontinence. The precise mechanism of action is unknown, although it is known to act centrally as an antidepressant. One potential route for peripheral action is through enhancement of sympathetic transmission, thereby reducing contractile tone in the bladder.
- Amitryptiline (tricyclic antidepressant) with inhibitory action at serotonin and noradrenaline reuptake sites: in contrast to duloxetine, it has significant antimuscarinic activity. Its action for the treatment of nocturnal enuresis is likely to be multi-fold, not only reducing parasympathetic tone, but also enhancing sympathetic relaxation, in the bladder. It can also relieve the depression which often accompanies nocturnal enuresis. Lastly, the antimuscarinic profile is associated with drowsiness, and so administration of the drug in the evening produces additional benefit.
- Desmopressin, a synthetic analogue of arginine vasopressin, is also used as a treatment of nocturnal enuresis, acting in the kidneys to reduce urinary formation.

The acute retention of urine can be extremely painful and is most commonly relieved through catheterisation. Where there is no bladder obstruction giving rise to urinary retention, bethanechol (a muscarinic agonist) or distigmine (a cholinesterase inhibitor) may be given to stimulate detrusor activity.

- In the case of benign prostatic hyperplasia (BPH), a common condition in elderly males, the growth of the prostate compresses the urethra, preventing ready drainage of the bladder. The obstruction may give rise to urinary stasis and an increased likelihood of urinary tract infections.
- α-Adrenoceptor antagonists, such as doxazosin and tamsulosin, act to relax the prostatic smooth muscle and reduce the obstruction, thereby allowing better drainage from the bladder.
- 5α-Reductase inhibitors, such as finasteride (see Chapter 33), reduce the formation of dihydrotestosterone, which stimulates the progression of some forms of BPH.
- Commonly, patients suffering from BPH undergo surgical removal of part of the prostate through the urethra (transurethral resection of the prostate: TURP).

KeyPoints (Figure 14.4)

- Diuretics are important cardiovascular drugs used to manage hypertension (thiazides) and chronic heart failure (loop diuretics and thiazides).
- Loop diuretics have powerful effects by reducing the ability of the loop of Henle to produce concentrated urine.
- Thiazide and loop diuretics both cause K^+ loss (hypokalaemia).
- Potassium-sparing diuretics are weak diuretics but reduce K^+ loss by either antagonism of MR receptors (e.g. spironolactone) or blocking sodium channels (e.g. amiloride).
- Antimuscarinic agents reduce bladder contractions to reduce urinary incontinence, particularly in the elderly.

Figure 14.4 Schematic diagram of a nephron showing the principal sites of diuretic action.

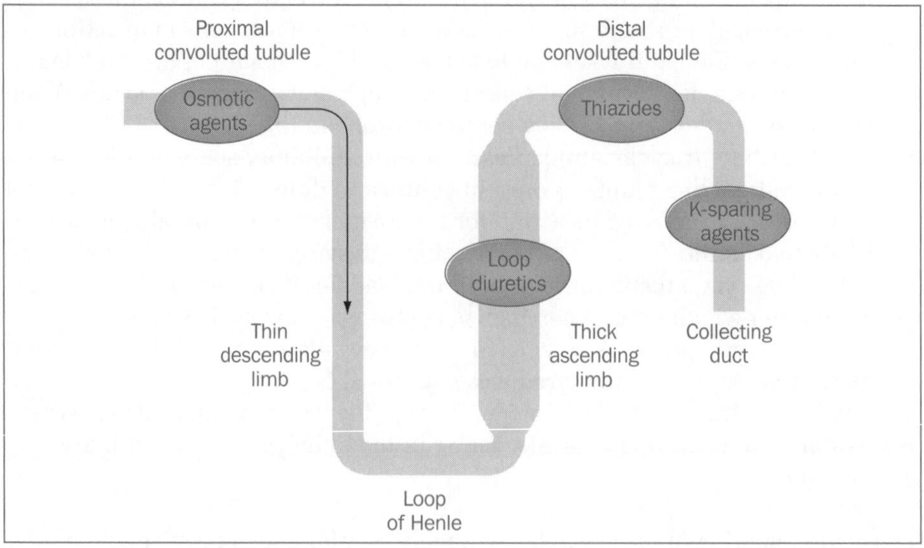

Self-assessment

1. **Which of the following cause K⁺ loss (hypokalaemia)?**
a. loop diuretics, such as furosemide
b. thiazides, such as bendroflumethiazide
c. mineralocorticoid receptor antagonists, such as spironolactone
d. ACE inhibitors, such as ramipril

2. **Which of the following are true or false regarding the actions of diuretics?**
a. Thiazides inhibit $3Na^+/2K^+$ ATPase (sodium pump)
b. Loop diuretics inhibit apical sodium channels
c. Amiloride blocks sodium channels in the DCT
d. Mineralocorticoid receptor antagonists (e.g. spironolactone) inhibit renin release

3. **Which of the following are true regarding the use of diuretics?**
a. Thiazides are often used in the management of hypertension
b. Thiazides may become ineffective in renal impairment
c. Loop diuretics are often used in the management of chronic heart failure
d. Potassium-sparing diuretics have weak diuretic effects

chapter 15
Antithrombotic agents: anticoagulants and antiplatelet drugs

Drugs that interfere with thrombosis are anticoagulants and antiplatelet drugs. Anticoagulants are used largely to prevent venous thrombosis (e.g. deep-vein thrombosis) and antiplatelet drugs are used to prevent arterial thrombosis (e.g. heart attacks and strokes).

Oral anticoagulants

e.g. warfarin

Mechanism of action
- Warfarin is a vitamin K antagonist and interferes with the synthesis of coagulation factors.
- Vitamin K is essential for production of prothrombin and factors VII, IX and X (vitamin K is important for posttranslational carboxylation of glutamic acid residues of these proteins).
- Warfarin blocks vitamin K reductase, needed for vitamin K to act as a cofactor in the synthesis of coagulation factors.

Adverse effects
- Many drug interactions.
- May lead to increased bleeding.

Clinical context
- Used to prevent thrombosis (after surgery, in patients with replaced heart valves, atrial fibrillation, pulmonary embolism, deep-vein thrombosis).
- Takes several days to act as it impairs the synthesis of new coagulation factors.
- Only works in vivo.
- Monitored by international normalised ratio (INR) (prothrombin time) with a specific target value and the dose is adjusted accordingly.
- Always used with caution due to the risk of interactions and bleeding.

Injectable anticoagulants

e.g. unfractionated heparin or low-molecular-weight heparins (LMWHs)

Mechanism of action
- Activate antithrombin III (natural protein).
- Antithrombin III inactivates some clotting factors and thrombin by complexing with serine protease activities of these factors.

Clinical context
- Immediate action.
- Inhibits coagulation both in vivo and in vitro.
- Used to prevent thrombosis (venous, unstable angina) and to prevent blood clotting on collection.

Thrombin inhibitors
- Dabigatran is a new drug and acts via inhibition of thrombin in the coagulation cascade.
- Thrombin inhibitors have fewer interactions and their actions appear more predictable.

Antiplatelet drugs

Low-dose aspirin
Mechanism of action (Figure 15.1)

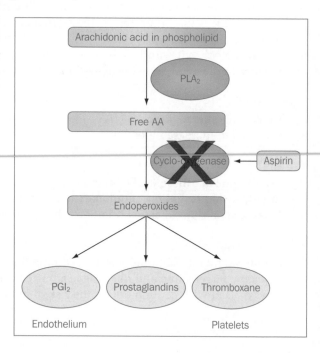

Figure 15.1 The mechanism of action of aspirin causing inhibition of cyclooxygenase, inhibiting the production of thromboxane (in platelets) and prostacyclin (PGI$_2$ on the endothelium). PLA$_2$, phospholipase A$_2$; AA, arachidonic acid.

- Low-dose aspirin inhibits cyclooxygenase (COX) irreversibly via acetylation of the *N*-terminal serine residue (see Chapter 7).
- It inhibits the production of both thromboxane (TXA_2) (which causes platelet aggregation and adhesion) from platelets and prostacyclin (PGI_2) (which prevents platelet aggregation) from endothelial cells.
- Platelets have no nuclei and so cannot produce any more cyclooxygenase so no more TXA_2 is produced until new platelets are synthesised (in about 7 days).
- Endothelial cells have nuclei and so can produce more COX (in a few hours) and PGI_2 is produced.
- Low-dose aspirin shifts the balance in favour of PGI_2 over TXA_2 and this reduces platelet aggregation.
- Higher doses of aspirin might adversely affect PGI_2 levels as endothelial COX activity would be inhibited for longer.

Adverse effects
- Low-dose aspirin is associated with gastric bleeding (see Chapter 9).

Clinical context
- Low-dose aspirin is effective at reducing heart attacks and thromboembolic strokes.

Dipyridamole
Mechanism of action
- Phosphodiesterase (PDE) inhibitor, preventing the breakdown of cyclic adenosine monophosphate (cAMP).
- cAMP is the second messenger for PGI_2, which inhibits platelet aggregation.
- Inhibits adenosine reuptake with higher affinity than PDE, leading to activation of adenosine receptors on the platelet surface, which act in the same way as prostacyclin receptors to prevent aggregation.

Clinical context
- Used to prevent thrombosis.
- Often used in conjunction with aspirin.

Glycoprotein IIb/IIIa
- Adenosine diphosphate (ADP) from aggregating platelets leads to expression of glycoprotein IIb/IIIa (GP IIb/IIIa).
- GP IIb/IIIa binds fibrinogen, which leads to cross-linking of platelets
- Clopidogrel is an ADP ($P2Y_{12}$) receptor antagonist and inhibits ADP-induced expression of GP IIb/IIIa.
- Clopidogrel is equally effective as low-dose aspirin and is often used when aspirin cannot be tolerated (e.g. aspirin-associated asthma).
- Abciximab is a monoclonal antibody against GP IIb/IIIa and is used by specialists.

Fibrinolytic (thrombolytic) agents ('clot busters')
e.g. streptokinase

Mechanism of action

- Fibrinolytic agents lead to activation of plasminogen to form plasmin.
- Plasminogen/plasmin is a natural mechanism to dissolve clots once they have formed.
- Plasmin digests the fibrin of the clot (and also some of the clotting factors) to dissolve clots once they have formed.

Adverse effects

- Fibrinolytic agents may dissolve normal clots (e.g. from surgery, peptic ulcers, haemorrhagic stroke), leading to bleeding. Patient's medical history is identified to avoid this.
- Streptokinase is immunogenic, which may lead to failure of treatment on re-exposure or an allergic response (due to antibody production).

Clinical context

- Given immediately after a heart attack to dissolve thrombus and lead to reperfusion.
- Some agents may be used in thromboembolic stroke.

KeyPoints

- Anticoagulants (warfarin and heparins) are more effective against venous thrombosis and antiplatelet drugs are more effective against arterial thrombosis.
- Warfarin is a vitamin K antagonist which impairs the production of new coagulation factors.
- Heparins act immediately via activation of antithrombin III.
- Low-dose aspirin is a COX inhibitor and favours PGI_2 over TXA_2.

Self-assessment

a. low-dose aspirin
b. warfarin
c. heparin
d. clopidogrel
e. thrombolytic agents
f. none of the above

Match the six options above to the following statements. An option may be used more than once:
1. This drug acts via inhibition of cyclooxygenase.
2. This drug blocks plasmin.
3. This drug is a vitamin K antagonist.
4. This drug is an ADP ($P2Y_{12}$) receptor antagonist.
5. This drug favours PGI_2 over TXA_2.
6. This drug is a TXA_2 receptor antagonist.
7. This drug inhibits coagulation in a test tube.

chapter 16
Antiobesity drugs

Obesity (body mass index > 30) is reaching epidemic proportions and is a major risk factor for the development of cardiovascular disease and diabetes. Obesity is invariably due to consumption of calories in excess of expenditure and is best managed by diet. In high-risk patients, diet may be used in conjunction with drug treatment and this approach leads to a 5–10% weight reduction. Two drugs are in use (orlistat and sibutramine):

Orlistat
- Orlistat inhibits the pancreatic lipases which digest fats. The fats are undigested and are not absorbed.
- The malabsorption of fat reduces calorie intake and leads to oily diarrhoea (steatorrhoea).
- Steatorrhoea means that patients will avoid high-fat foods to prevent this unpleasant adverse effect.

Sibutramine
- Centrally acting.
- 5-Hydroxytryptamine and noradrenaline reuptake inhibitor which acts in the hypothalamus and suppresses appetite.
- It is associated with increasing blood pressure due to enhanced sympathetic activity.

Rimonabant
- This is a cannabinoid CB_1 receptor antagonist.
- Rimonabant acts both centrally to suppress endogenous cannabinoid-induced appetite and peripherally. It has been shown to be of benefit in patients with metabolic disorders, including diabetes. However, it is associated with central nervous system side-effects such as depression and its use was suspended in 2008.

KeyPoints

- Drugs should be used alongside diet and exercise.
- Orlistat is a pancreatic lipase inhibitor.
- Sibutramine is a 5-hydroxytryptamine/noradrenaline reuptake inhibitor.

chapter 17
Asthma and chronic obstructive pulmonary disease

Asthma is a common condition with reversible increases in airway resistance, involving bronchoconstriction and inflammation. It is characterised by reversible decreases in the FEV_1:FVC ratio (less than 70–80% suggests increased airway resistance). It may be managed pharmacologically by bronchodilators and anti-inflammatory drugs.

Chronic obstructive pulmonary disease (COPD) is a combination of chronic bronchitis and emphysema. In chronic bronchitis, there is increased mucus, airway obstruction and intercurrent infections. In emphysema there is destruction of alveoli. In COPD, FEV_1 is reduced with little variation or reversibility and there is a strong association with smoking.

Autonomic control of airways

Parasympathetic
Acetylcholine acts on muscarinic M_3 receptors to cause bronchoconstriction and increased mucus.

Sympathetic
There is little or no direct innervation. Circulating adrenaline acts on β_2-adrenoceptors on bronchial smooth muscle to cause relaxation.

Asthma

- There is often a genetic predisposition and an attack may be provoked by:
  - allergens
  - cold air
  - viral infections
  - smoking
  - exercise.
- The attack may have an early (immediate) phase due to bronchoconstriction and this may be followed several hours later by a late phase due to inflammatory mediator release.

- Mediators include histamine, prostaglandins, leukotrienes, platelet-activating factor and interleukins and involves leukocytes (especially eosinophils and mononuclear cells).
- Asthma is characterised by ongoing inflammation of the airways with hypersensitivity of the sensory nerves.
- Troublesome cough is common.

Bronchodilators

β_2-adrenoceptor agonists
e.g. salbutamol (Ventolin)

Mechanism of action
- Act on β_2-adrenoceptors on smooth muscle to increase cyclic adenosine monophosphate (cAMP) to cause bronchodilatation.

Clinical context
- Given by inhalation.
- Agents of first choice for asthma and COPD.
- Cause rapid relaxation of the airways.
- Prolonged use may lead to desensitisation and receptor downregulation.

Long-acting β-agonists (LABA)
e.g. salmeterol

These act in a similar way to short-acting β_2-adrenoceptor agonists but have a more prolonged action due to binding near to the receptor (an exosite) and being retained locally.

Clinical context
- Have a slow rate for onset of actions and so are not used to relieve an attack.
- Given for long-term prevention and long-term control (e.g. overnight).

Xanthines
e.g. theophylline

Mechanism of action
- Possibly act via phosphodiesterase inhibition, leading to increased cAMP levels and relaxation.
- They also act as adenosine receptor antagonists, which may contribute to the antiasthma profile.

Adverse effects
- They have a narrow therapeutic window and toxicity leads to nausea, tachycardia and convulsions.

Clinical context

- Aminophylline is a salt which yields theophylline.
- Xanthines are given orally (theophylline, aminophylline) or intravenously (aminophylline).
- They are used orally in asthma and intravenously to manage severe asthma attacks.

Muscarinic receptor antagonists

e.g. ipratropium/tiotropium

Mechanism of action

- Competitive antagonism of bronchial muscarinic receptors.
- Block parasympathetic bronchoconstriction.

Clinical context

- Given by inhalation to limit antimuscarinic side-effects.
- Of limited value in asthma, but widely used in COPD.

Anti-inflammatory agents

Corticosteroids

e.g. beclometasone (inhalation), prednisolone (oral)

Mechanism of action (see Chapter 33 for molecular mechanism)

- Anti-inflammatory by activation of intracellular receptors, leading to altered gene transcription (decreased cytokine production) and production of lipocortin, which inhibits phospholipase A_2 and the release of arachidonic acid.

Adverse effects

- Inhalation limits systemic effects associated with steroid use (e.g. adrenal suppression, susceptibility to infection.
- Inhalation may lead to local effects (e.g. throat infections, hoarseness).

Clinical context

- Beneficial effects via alterations in gene transcription take several days to take effect.
- Corticosteroids are used to prevent asthma attacks but will not relieve them.
- They are central to the management of asthma and an additional action may be to prevent desensitisation of β_2-adrenoceptors by β_2-agonists.
- They may be of benefit in a small proportion of COPD patients.

Leukotriene receptor antagonists (LTRAs)

e.g. montelukast

- Antagonise actions of leukotrienes at $CysLT_1$ receptors which cause bronchoconstriction and inflammation.
- Used in asthma for both prevention and bronchodilatation.

Cromones

e.g. sodium cromoglicate

- Uncertain mechanism of action but may stabilise mast cells, reduce the release of platelet-activating factor and cytokines and reduce reflexes of sensory nerves.
- Used to prevent asthmatic attacks.
- Weakly effective but lacking side-effects.

Drugs causing bronchoconstriction

β-blockers

- β-blockers (including cardioselective β_1-blockers) may block adrenaline acting at bronchial β_2-adrenoceptors and cause bronchospasm.
- β-blockers are avoided in patients with asthma. If one is essential, then a more cardioselective β_1-blocker is used with extreme caution.
- In COPD β-blockers are avoided unless benefits outweigh the disadvantages, in which case a cardioselective β_1-blocker should be used.

Non-steroidal anti-inflammatory drugs (NSAIDs)

- In a proportion of patients with asthma, NSAIDs may provoke asthma.
- This is thought to be due to cyclooxygenase inhibition leading to arachidonic acid being diverted to increased leukotriene production.

KeyPoints

- Drugs are relievers (e.g. β_2-adrenoceptor agonists) or preventers (e.g. corticosteroids).
- β-blockers and NSAIDs can cause bronchoconstriction.

Self-assessment

1. **Which of the following mediators may be involved in an asthma attack?**
a. histamine
b. adenosine
c. adrenaline
d. leukotrienes

2. **Which one of the following best describes the action of β_2-agonists?**
a. anti-inflammatory
b. simulation of β_2-adrenoceptors coupled to increased potassium conductance
c. blockade of circulating adrenaline
d. simulation of β_2-adrenoceptors coupled to an increase in cAMP

3. **Which of the following are true or false regarding xanthines (such as theophylline)?**
a. likely enhance the effects of β_2-agonists
b. drugs of first choice in COPD

c. drugs with a narrow therapeutic window
d. phosphodiesterase activators

4. **Which of the following are associated with causing asthma attacks in susceptible patients?**
a. corticosteroids
b. β-blockers
c. NSAIDs
d. exercise

chapter 18
Allergy

An allergic response is an immune response to foreign substances or allergens. Specific immunity produces specific and highly amplified responses to prior exposure and in type 1 hypersensitivity the allergen leads to cross-linking of immunoglobulin E (IgE) by allergen and mast cell degranulation and release of mediators of inflammation (with increased permeability, chemotaxis, mucus and oedema). Mediators include histamine, prostanoids, leukotrienes and bradykinin (see Chapter 7).

Allergic rhinitis, including hayfever and dermatitis, are common allergic responses. Allergic rhinitis includes nasal itching, runny nose, sneezing and sore eyes and is in response to allergens such as pollen and house dust mite. Certain drugs can cause allergic reactions, e.g. penicillins.

Antihistamines

e.g. loratadine, cetirizine (both non-sedating) and chlorphenamine (sedating)

Mechanism of action
- Histamine H_1 receptor antagonists block the actions of histamine associated with the symptoms.

Adverse effects
- Sedating agents may penetrate the blood–brain barrier, causing drowsiness.
- Some older agents (e.g. promethazine) have antimuscarinic side-effects.

Clinical context
- Sedating and non-sedating agents are equally effective and so newer, non-sedating agents are preferred.
- They are given orally to relieve symptoms of hayfever and more systemic allergic responses (e.g. penicillin allergy).
- Topical agents are available for application to eyes, nose and skin (although they are not recommended for skin).

Topical corticosteroids

e.g. beclometasone, budesonide
- Available as over-the-counter topical medicines for moderate/persistent nasal symptoms in hayfever.
- Have anti-inflammatory actions.
- Are very effective.

- Topical application limits systemic side-effects.
- Take several days for an effect.

Cromones
e.g. sodium cromoglicate and nedocromil sodium
- Available as eye drops for conjunctival symptoms.
- See Chapter 17.

Decongestants

e.g. topical (xylometazoline, oxymetazoline) and oral (phenylephrine, pseudoephedrine, phenylpropanolamine)

Mechanism of action
- Xylometazoline, oxymetazoline and phenylephrine are α-adrenoceptor agonists which cause local vasoconstriction and reduce mucus flow.
- Pseudoephedrine and phenylpropanolamine are largely indirectly acting sympathomimetic agents which cause the release of noradrenaline, leading to vasoconstriction, including in the nose.

Adverse effects
- Oral agents have sympathetic activity and so should not be used in untreated hypertension, hyperthyroidism, diabetes and ischaemic heart disease.
- Prolonged use of topical agents is associated with rebound congestion.

Clinical context
- Decongestants are widely used for runny noses in allergy and colds.
- Topical agents are more effective and cause fewer systemic side-effects.

Leukotriene receptor antagonists

e.g. montelukast
  See Chapter 17. They may help with hayfever.

Anaphylaxis

Anaphylaxis is a severe, life-threatening allergic response with massive mediator release (including histamine). There may be swollen lips, eyelids, bronchospasm and hypotension. Treatment includes oxygen, adrenaline, antihistamines and corticosteroids.

Adrenaline

Adrenaline is used in the emergency treatment of anaphylaxis. It is given by injection to cause bronchodilation (via β_2-adrenoceptors) and increase cardiac output (via β_1-adrenoceptors).

KeyPoints

- Antihistamines have a key role as histamine H_1 receptor antagonists.
- Corticosteroids also have a key role (see Chapter 33).

Self-assessment

Which of the following are true or false regarding antihistamines?
1. They are histamine H_2 receptor antagonists.
2. They are all sedating.
3. They are histamine H_1 receptor antagonists.
4. Non-sedating agents are equally as effective as sedating agents.

chapter 19
Anxiolytics and hypnotics

Anxiety, involving feelings of apprehension and worry, is a normal reaction to stress, but if the responses are inappropriate or excessive, this might be regarded as an anxiety disorder needing treatment. Anxiety disorder is a component of a number of broader conditions, including psychosis and depression, and is accompanied by somatic symptoms such as palpitations, sweating, nausea, headache and other pain. Sleep disturbances are a common feature of anxiety disorders and can be treated largely with the same anxiolytic drugs (then referred to as hypnotics). Physiological anxiety, such as that experienced during bereavement, should not be drug-treated since this might inhibit the coping process. The formerly used term 'minor tranquilliser' should not be used interchangeably with 'anxiolytic', not least because the effects of these drugs are by no means minor. The key to successful drug treatment of anxiety disorder is to use the smallest dose for the shortest possible time.

Benzodiazepines

e.g. diazepam, alprazolam, chlordiazepoxide, flurazepam, lorazepam, oxazepam, nitrazepam, temazepam

Mechanism of action
- Benzodiazepines potentiate inhibitory neurotransmission in the brain by increasing γ-aminobutyric acid (GABA) binding to the $GABA_A$ receptor via interaction with an allosteric site.

Adverse effects
- Contraindicated in respiratory depression and hepatic impairment; should not be used for chronic psychosis or alone for treatment of depression.
- Caution indicated if there is muscle weakness (e.g. myasthenia gravis), history of substance abuse or personality disorder.
- Drowsiness, confusion, amnesia, hangover.
- Paradoxical increase in aggression.
- Dependence with associated abstinence syndrome, particularly for shorter-acting drugs (lorazepam, oxazepam). Withdrawal must be gradual.

Clinical context
- Used for short-term treatment of anxiety or insomnia.
- Usually administered orally but occasionally (diazepam, lorazepam) by intravenous injection for control of acute panic attack.

- Nitrazepam and lorazepam have prolonged duration of action and are used as hypnotics, although hangover effects are possible; shorter-acting lorazepam and temazepam have no such residual actions.

Buspirone
Mechanism of action
- Modulates serotonin neurotransmission by acting on presynaptic $5HT_{1A}$ receptors.

Adverse effects
- Contraindicated in epilepsy.
- Nausea, dizziness, headache, excitement.

Clinical context
- As effective as benzodiazepines (eventually) but better tolerated.
- Takes weeks of treatment to show efficacy; acute anxiety may require benzodiazepine co-administration until buspirone takes effect.

β-blockers

e.g. propranolol, oxprenolol

β-blockers reduce the sympathetic autonomic symptoms of anxiety disorder, such as palpitations and tremor, which can be of value, although they have no effect on psychological components.

Antidepressants as anxiolytics

Some antidepressants are licensed for the treatment of chronic generalised anxiety disorder (e.g. paroxetine, venlafaxine). As with treatment of depression, anxiolytic effects take weeks to develop and co-treatment with a benzodiazepine might be indicated.

KeyPoints

- Drug treatment of anxiety disorder should be as short as possible and use the lowest possible dose.
- Benzodiazepines are effective, rapidly acting anxiolytics and hypnotics but have the potential to cause dependence.
- Buspirone is an effective anxiolytic, although it is slow to act.
- β-blockers are helpful in combating somatic effects in anxiety.
- Some antidepressants are a reasonable choice for treating chronic anxiety.

Self-assessment

In the management of anxiety, which of the following are true or false?

1. Insomnia and anxiety are largely treated with the same drugs.
2. Benzodiazepines block GABA receptors.
3. Lorazepam has a longer duration of action than nitrazepam.
4. Longer-acting benzodiazepines are more liable to cause dependence.
5. Benzodiazepines can cause aggression.
6. Buspirone is a $5HT_{1A}$ antagonist.
7. Buspirone's anxiolytic effects takes weeks to appear.
8. Oxprenolol is as effective an anxiolytic as diazepam.
9. Anxiolytics can be used to treat depression.
10. Barbiturates are old-fashioned, yet sometimes useful anxiolytics.

chapter 20
Antidepressants

- Depression is a long-standing condition associated with feelings of low self-esteem, a lack of motivation, an inability to derive pleasure and sleep disturbance, often with early waking. There is a risk of suicide.
- The disorder might be accompanied by anxiety, panic, obsession and phobia.
- Bipolar disorder (manic depression) involves periods of low mood alternating with manic behaviour (excessive enthusiasm, self-confidence, grandiose delusions, increased libido, aggression and impatience).
- Depression has a close association with chronic illnesses (e.g. multiple sclerosis, myocardial infarction, stroke, Parkinson's disease, cancer, human immunodeficiency virus (HIV)) and untreated depression can compromise treatment of comorbidities. Drug misuse can also complicate diagnosis and therapy.
- The cause is probably multifactorial and may be precipitated by major life events such as childbirth or bereavement.
- Genetic links are probable but no causal gene(s) have been unequivocally identified.
- The monoamine theory of depression proposes that depression is due to a deficiency of monoamine neurotransmitters (noradrenaline, 5-hydroxytryptamine (5HT)) somewhere in the brain. Other suggestions include possible overactivity of the hypothalamic–pituitary–adrenal (stress) axis causing excessive circulating corticosteroids and neuronal death.

Serotonin-selective reuptake inhibitors (SSRIs)

e.g. citalopram, fluoxetine, paroxetine, sertraline

Mechanism of action
- Selective inhibition of neuronal reuptake and enhancement of synaptic concentrations of 5HT.

Adverse effects
- SSRIs have fewer side-effects than tricyclic antidepressants (TCAs). They are less dangerous in overdose than TCAs or monoamine oxidase inhibitors (MAOIs) but are still associated with gastrointestinal disturbances (nausea), weight change (loss or gain), rashes, sexual dysfunction, abnormal dreams and sleep disturbances.
- SSRIs may be associated with a withdrawal reaction (especially paroxetine).

Clinical context

- Commonly first-line therapy for moderate to major depression.
- Take 2–4 weeks to have an effect in depression.
- Some SSRIs are also used in anxiety.
- Only fluoxetine is suitable for treatment of under-18-year-olds and, as with other SSRIs, there is a small risk of self-harm and suicidal thoughts.

Tricyclic antidepressants

e.g. amitriptyline, dothiepin, imipramine, lofepramine, nortriptyline, clomipramine

Mechanism of action

- Inhibition of neuronal uptake of noradrenaline and 5HT.
- Antagonism of neurotransmitter receptors, including muscarinic, histamine and 5HT, contributes to side-effects.

Adverse effects

- Possess antimuscarinic activity, which causes side-effects such as dry mouth, blurred vision, constipation, urinary retention.
- TCAs vary in the degree of sedation caused; might be helpful for sleep disturbances or unwelcome. Amitriptyline and dothiepin are sedative; imipramine, lofepramine and nortriptyline are less sedating.
- TCAs have adverse cardiac effects, e.g. prolonged QT interval on electrocardiogram; increase in catecholamines predisposes to heart block and arrhythmias. Cardiac effects (except lofepramine) and enhancement of alcohol effects (respiratory depression) mean that these agents are dangerous in overdose.
- Should not be combined with other antidepressants (serious adverse interaction).

Clinical context

- TCAs are generally used in depression when SSRIs are ineffective.
- Sedating ones may be used when sleep is disturbed.
- Beneficial effects take 2–4 weeks in depression.

Monoamine oxidase inhibitors

e.g. isocarboxazid, moclobemide, phenelzine, tranylcypromine

Mechanism of action

- Inhibition of enzyme (MAO) that metabolises monoamines.

Adverse effects

- MAO blockade prevents breakdown of monoamine transmitters and the indirectly acting sympathomimetic amine, tyramine, present in the diet, e.g. in cheese, causing danger of hypertensive crisis. Older MAOIs inhibit irreversibly; reactions may persist for 2–3 weeks after treatment has stopped until new enzyme synthesised. Other side-effects include postural hypotension, headache, dizziness, sexual dysfunction.

- MAO-A metabolises mainly noradrenaline and 5HT; phenylethylamine is the preferred substrate for MAO-B. Tyramine and dopamine are metabolised by both. To reduce side-effects and interactions, second-generation selective inhibitors of MAO have been developed.

Clinical context

- Not widely used any more but might be worth trying in patients refractory to other drugs.
- Moclobemide, a selective reversible inhibitor of MAO-A (RIMA), reduces interaction with food. Moclobemide is relatively well tolerated with few sexual side-effects; action reverses in 24–48 hours.

Selective noradrenaline reuptake inhibitors (NARIs)

e.g. reboxetine
- Limited side-effects (urinary problems, nausea, dry mouth, constipation possible).
- Not recommended for under-18s and elderly.

Serotonin/noradrenaline reuptake inhibitors (SNRIs)

e.g. venlafaxine
- SSRI-like action in initial 75 mg dose range. Anecdotally greater efficacy and faster onset compared with SSRIs (unproven).
- Dose-dependent risk of increased blood pressure; contraindicated in patients with cardiac arrhythmias or uncontrolled hypertension.
- Side-effect profile similar to SSRIs.
- Mirtazapine has α_2-adrenoceptor antagonist activity. Inhibiting negative feedback by these presynaptic receptors increases noradrenaline and 5HT transmission. Sedation predominates in early treatment but antimuscarinic effects are limited.

Other drugs

Lithium

- Lithium (usually as lithium carbonate) is first-line therapy for the prophylaxis of bipolar disorder.
- Lithium is toxic in overdose, so need to monitor blood levels regularly (every 3 months once stable) to keep within narrow therapeutic window of 0.4–1 mmol/l (serum) 12 h after a dose. Mechanism of action uncertain (see Chapter 3).
- Antipsychotic drugs (haloperidol, prochlorperazine) are quick-acting and safer alternatives in the treatment of acute manic phase. Carbamazepine can

be used for bipolar disorder prophylaxis, particularly in patients with rapid cycling illness (four or more episodes per year).

St John's wort

- Preparations of St John's wort (*Hypericum perforatum*) are widely available in health food shops, but not licensed in the UK as a medicine.
- St John's wort inhibits reuptake of 5HT, noradrenaline and dopamine and is a weak MAOI (properties, including side-effects, resemble first-generation antidepressants).
- There are pharmacokinetic interactions due to enzyme induction. Care is needed with anticonvulsants, ciclosporin, digoxin, anti-HIV drugs, oral contraceptives, SSRIs, theophylline and warfarin.
- Active ingredients are not fully characterised and differ from preparation to preparation. Self-medication with unlicensed remedies can divert patients away from professional care and should be avoided.

Tryptophan

- Amino acid precursor of 5HT, occasionally prescribed. Enhances central 5HT synthesis, supporting the monoamine theory of depression.

Tianeptine (Stablon)

- Paradoxically, enhances 5HT reuptake, casting doubt on the simple monoamine theory.
- Not licensed in the UK.

General features of antidepressant drug therapy

- There is no significant difference in efficacy between new and old antidepressants. Approximately 50–65% patients will be much improved if they take antidepressants compared with 25–30% on placebo (National Institute for Health and Clinical Excellence 2004).
- All drugs take some weeks to work and patients may initially feel worse.
- Failure of treatment (typically after 4 weeks) would indicate another drug should be used.
- Some antidepressant drugs have relatively long half-lives (e.g. fluoxetine, 7–9 days) and in the case of irreversible MAOIs it could take more than a month to synthesise new enzyme, particularly in the elderly. An alternative drug should not be started until it is certain that the first has been cleared.
- Treatment should continue for at least 6 months after recovery to prevent relapse (common) and treatment should not be abruptly withdrawn.

Reference

National Institute for Health and Clinical Excellence (2004) *Depression: Management of Depression in Primary and Secondary Care*. National clinical practice guideline number 23. London: National Institute for Health and Clinical Excellence.

KeyPoints

- Depression is a long-standing, relapsing illness requiring long-term therapy.
- SSRIs are the usual first-line therapy because they are associated with less severe side-effects than first-generation TCAs and MAOIs; they are no more effective.
- There is a significant lag time before antidepressants produce clinical benefit.
- Therapy must continue for a significant period after remission to prevent relapse.

Self-assessment

1. **Which of the following drugs inhibits 5HT reuptake?**
a. citalopram
b. reboxetine
c. St John's wort
d. venlafaxine

2. **Which of the following could be used to treat the acute manic phase of bipolar disorder?**
a. lithium
b. mirtazapine
c. prochlorperazine
d. carbamazepine

3. **Which of the following statements are correct?**
a. Depression is due to a deficiency of monoamine neurotransmitters in the brain
b. SSRIs are more effective than MAOIs
c. Changing from one antidepressant to another is pointless
d. Antidepressant drugs have short half-lives

4. **Which of the following are side-effects of TCAs?**
a. urinary retention
b. hypotension
c. constipation
d. ECG abnormalities

5. **Combination of MAOIs should be avoided with which of the following?**
a. TCAs
b. strong cheese
c. paracetamol
d. over-the-counter cold remedies

chapter 21
Antiepileptic drugs

- A seizure is an episode of abnormal synchronised electrical activity in the brain leading to acute changes in the brain and muscles. Individuals may suffer a single seizure, due to a variety of causes, without any recurrence.
- Epilepsy is a condition in which there is a tendency to suffer recurrent seizures.
- A partial seizure starts with a focus of electrical activity in a small part of the brain which spreads to other parts. In a simple partial seizure, symptoms vary according to the focus (involuntary movements, paraesthesia (prickling of skin), flashing lights) but with no loss of consciousness.
- In a complex partial seizure (temporal-lobe epilepsy), abnormal activity starts in the temporal lobe (hippocampus or amygdala) or frontal lobe and there is altered consciousness (loss of grip on reality). A complex partial seizure involves involuntary movements and impaired memory of seizure, and is often preceded by an aura (change in emotion or specific sensation, e.g. odd taste or smell).
- A generalised seizure does not start from a defined focus and involves both cerebral hemispheres.
- A myoclonic seizure is generalised and consists of brief repetitive, rhythmic jerks that could involve a single muscle group or all parts of the body.
- An absence seizure (petit mal) is generalised and involves a sudden brief interruption in attention or consciousness. Sufferers have a blank stare and occasionally minor motor symptoms (blinking, lip smacking). There is no aura.
- A tonic-clonic (grand mal) seizure is generalised and involves stiffening or rigidity of the entire body followed by rhythmic movements of the limbs. There will be a loss of consciousness, preceded by an aura.
- Medicated patients suffering from epilepsy are allowed to drive a private motor vehicle providing they have been seizure-free for 1 year or if they have only suffered seizures during sleep for a period of 3 years.

Antiepileptic drugs

Mechanism of action
- Abnormal neuronal excitability can be reduced in a number of ways (Table 21.1) and antiepileptic drugs have multiple actions on different ion channels, i.e. their effects are pleiotropic.

Table 21.1 Antiepileptic drugs indicated for different seizure types

Seizure type	Absence	Myoclonic	Partial, with or without secondary generalisation	Generalised tonic/clonic
First-line drug(s)	Ethosuximide Valproate	Valproate	Carbamazepine Lamotrigine Topiramate Oxcarbazepine	Carbamazepine Lamotrigine Topiramate Valproate
Other drugs	Clonazepam Lamotrigine	Clobazam Clonazepa	Clobazam Gabapentin Phenytoin	Oxcarbazepine Valproate

- Major molecular targets are:
  - Sodium channels: drugs prolong the inactivated state of the channel and halt action potential propagation. Sodium channel inhibitors show specificity for treatment of partial and secondarily generalised seizures.
  - T-type Ca^{2+} channels. These are normally depolarised and inactive in the awake state. In absence seizures, hyperpolarisation is thought to activate the channel and generate action potentials. Drugs inhibiting T-channels (e.g. ethosuximide) are specifically used for absence seizures.
  - Voltage-operated Ca^{2+} (VOC) channels: control Ca^{2+} entry into neuronal terminals and regulate neurotransmitter release.
  - Activation of γ-aminobutyric acid (GABA) system increases inhibitory tone.
  - Blockade of glutamate channels inhibits major excitatory system in brain.

Adverse effects
- Side-effects of antiepileptic drugs (particularly older agents) are common and potentially severe.
- Na^+ channel inhibitors can cause skin reactions, notably Stevens–Johnson syndrome, a life-threatening hypersensitivity condition in which cell death causes the epidermis to separate from the dermis. They can also induce a wide variety of serious liver and blood disorders and patients should receive instructions on recognising the signs. Also, nausea, vomiting, gastrointestinal upsets, dizziness, confusion and visual disturbances are possible.
- Phenytoin can cause gingival hyperplasia, acne and hirsutism.
- Lamotrigine can induce sleep disturbances, hallucinations and occasional increases in seizure frequency.
- Ethosuximide can cause gastrointestinal disturbances, anorexia with weight loss, bone marrow suppression, Stevens–Johnson syndrome and systemic lupus erythematosus.
- GABA potentiators can cause ataxia, dizziness and fatigue.

- Since combinations of two or more drugs concurrently may be required to keep patients seizure-free, interactions between them must be considered. Interactions are generally due to hepatic enzyme induction or inhibition and are complex and unpredictable.
- Antiepileptic drugs are teratogenic to varying degrees and the management of epilepsy in pregnancy is a specialist area.

Clinical context

- The decision to start on antiepileptic drug therapy should be taken in consultation with the patient after discussions of risks/benefits, seizure type, prognosis, comorbidities and lifestyle with an epilepsy specialist.
- Some adults may decide not to embark on drug therapy.
- Initiation of therapy would usually only follow a second seizure unless a neurological deficit, brain abnormality or definite epileptic activity on electroencephalogram is identified or the risks of seizure are unacceptable.
- The goal of treatment is to secure a seizure-free life, but a balance between minimum seizure frequency and drug tolerability can be a realistic objective.
- Monotherapy with an antiepileptic drug is preferable and, if the first is unsuccessful, monotherapy with a second should be attempted before combinations of drugs are tried. If the combination is not satisfactory, one drug should be tapered off before a third is tried.
- Newer antiepileptic drugs (lamotrigine, gabapentin, topiramate, tiagabine, oxcarbazepine, levetiracetam) are generally recommended due to their efficacy and fewer side-effects.
- Dosing frequency should be kept as low as is compatible with an appropriate plasma concentration; most drugs are given twice daily, but lamotrigine, for example, has a long half-life and can be given once a day at bedtime.
- Phenytoin shows zero-order kinetics (see Chapter 8). Dosing with phenytoin should be increased gradually with monitoring of plasma concentrations.
- Blood tests are only required if there is a specific clinical need, e.g. suspected toxicity or non-compliance with dosing regimen.
- Withdrawal from treatment should only be considered after 2 years of freedom from seizures and then over 2–3 months (6 months for benzodiazepines such as clonazepam). One drug at a time should be withdrawn in combination treatment regimes.

KeyPoints

- Epilepsy is a condition in which there is a tendency to suffer recurrent seizures.
- Seizures may be of the partial, generalised or absence types.
- Antiepileptic drugs have multiple actions on ion channels, reducing neuronal activity in the brain (Table 21.2).

continued

Table 21.2 Ion channel activity of antiepileptic drugs

	Na$^+$ channel inactivation	T-Ca^{2+} channel block	VOC Ca^{2+} channel block	GABA channel activation	Glutamate channel inhibition
Carbamazepine	X				
Valproate	X	X		X	
Lamotrigine	X		X		
Phenytoin	X				
Ethosuxamide		X			
Topiramate	X		X	X	X
Oxcarbazepine	X				
Clonazepam				X	
Clobazam				X	
Gabapentin			X		X

VOC, voltage-operated Ca^{2+} channel GABA, gamma-aminobutyric acid.

KeyPoints

- Drugs inhibit Na$^+$ channels, T-type and voltage-activated Ca^{2+} channels and glutamate receptor channels and enhance GABA channels.
- All drugs have significant side-effects and interactions that can limit their use. Pregnancy or risk of pregnancy is a key issue.
- Newer antiepileptic drugs are generally recommended.

Self-assessment

1. **Fill in the missing words:**
a. A(n) _____ seizure has a focal starting point in the brain.
b. A(n) _____ seizure has no focal point and begins in both cerebral hemispheres.
c. A(n) _____ seizure involves brief lapses of consciousness.
d. A(n) _____ seizure is generalised and involves stiffening or rigidity of the entire body followed by rhythmic movements of the limbs.

2. **Fill in the missing drug names:**
a. _____ is first-line therapy for absence seizures.
b. _____ is first-line therapy for myoclonic seizures.
c. _____ is first-line therapy for partial seizures.
d. _____ is first-line therapy for grand mal seizures.

3. **Answer true or false:**
a. Carbamazepine inactivates Na$^+$ channels.
b. Lamotrigine inactivates Na$^+$ channels.

c. Ethosuximide blocks glutamate receptor channels.
d. Clonazepam potentiates the effects of GABA.

4. Which of the following statements are true?
a. Lamotrigine can cause gingival hyperplasia, acne and hirsutism.
b. Skin hypersensitivity is a major side-effect of many antiepileptic drugs.
c. Epileptic patients cannot drive commercial motor vehicles.
d. Withdrawal from antiepileptic drugs should be considered after a seizure-free period of 1 year.

chapter 22
Antipsychotic drugs

- Psychosis is a blanket term for mental disorders in which thought and perception are severely impaired. They may include hallucinations, delusions, personality changes and disorganised thinking, resulting in a loss of contact with reality and an inability to cope with daily life.
- The most common form of psychosis is schizophrenia, in which sufferers experience delusions, hallucinations and thought disorders (referred to as positive symptoms) and social withdrawal, reduced emotional responses and dementia (negative symptoms).
- Incidence is about 1% in the UK population.
- A genetic component is strong but not inevitable.
- Schizophrenia often appears between 20 and 30 years but might start in the teenage years.
- It appears to be a developmental rather than degenerative disorder.
- About 20% of patients will never relapse after a single 'breakdown' but, typically, schizophrenia is characterised by repeated acute episodes.
- On the basis of mechanisms of effective drug treatments, schizophrenia is suggested to be due to overactivity of cortical dopamine-containing neurones. Amphetamine-induced psychosis resembles schizophrenia; amphetamine releases dopamine in the brain.

Antipsychotic drugs

- These are also known as neuroleptics and as major tranquillisers. This is inappropriate since the goal of treatment is to reduce disordered thoughts without a reduction in consciousness.
- They are relatively 'dirty' drugs with an affinity for a number of receptors.

Classification
- Phenothiazines, categorised into three groups:
  1. severely sedative with moderate extrapyramidal (movement disorder) and antimuscarinic effects, e.g. chlorpromazine
  2. moderately sedative with pronounced antimuscarinic but few extrapyramidal effects, e.g. pericyazine
  3. few sedative or antimuscarinic but marked extrapyramidal effects, e.g. fluphenazine, trifluoperazine
- Other 'typical' neuroleptics; butyrophenones, e.g. haloperidol; diphenylbutylpiperidines, e.g. pimozide; thioxanthines, e.g. flupentixol; substituted benzamides, e.g. sulpiride
- Atypical antipsychotics, e.g. amisulpride, clozapine, olanzapine, risperidone, zotepine.

Mechanism of action

- All neuroleptics antagonise dopamine D_2 receptors in the cerebral cortex. Coincident blockade of D_2 receptors in the nigrostriatal pathway leads to Parkinson's disease-like extrapyramidal side-effects.
- Neuroleptics, most notably the atypicals also, have affinity for other monoamine receptors, particularly the $5HT_2$ and dopamine D_4 receptors.

Adverse effects

- Movement disorders are the most serious. These comprise:
  - acute dystonias (involuntary movements, including muscle spasms and protruding tongue)
  - parkinsonian tremors, which appear in the first few weeks of treatment and often decline
  - akathisia (restlessness)
  - tardive dyskinesia. As the name suggests, tardive dyskinesia can appear months or even years after the start of treatment and can be disabling and practically irreversible. It consists of involuntary movements of limbs, face, tongue and trunk. The mechanism is not clear but likely involves enhancement of dopaminergic signalling in the basal ganglia in response to blockade by the neuroleptic.
- Atypical neuroleptics are less likely to cause tardive dyskinesia, but the reasons for this are unclear.
- Antimuscarinic effects include blurred vision, dry mouth and urinary retention.
- Antihistamine effects include sedation.
- There may be orthostatic hypotension due to α-adrenoceptor blockade.
- Weight gain may be due to 5-hydroxytryptamine (5HT) antagonism.
- Neuroleptic malignant syndrome is rare but comprises malignant hyperthermia with muscle rigidity and confusion. It is usually reversible but death can result from renal or cardiovascular system failure.
- Antipsychotics should be used with caution in patients with cardiovascular disease or with a history of epilepsy.
- Caution is also required in the elderly; olanzapine and risperidone are associated with increased risk of stroke in the elderly and should not be used for treating behavioural symptoms of dementia.
- Clozapine is associated with a significant incidence of neutropenia and blood count monitoring is required.

Clinical context

- A first, acute schizophrenic episode should be treated with an atypical antipsychotic (not clozapine).
- Atypical antipsychotic agents are considered to be associated with fewer side-effects than older agents and can be effective in those patients (about 30%) who are resistant to treatment with typical drugs.
- All antipsychotics are more effective against the positive than negative symptoms of schizophrenia.

- Clozapine should be prescribed if two other drugs (one an atypical), used sequentially for 6–8 weeks, have failed to be effective.
- Sedative drugs such as chlorpromazine are still used routinely, e.g. in violent patients, without causing stupor.
- Emergency intramuscular injection of an antipsychotic to control a severely disturbed patient should be at a lower dose than the corresponding oral dose of the same drug since first-pass metabolism is avoided.
- There is no need to change to an atypical drug if a typical agent is providing control of symptoms and not producing unacceptable side-effects.
- Doses should be titrated upwards slowly (not more than once weekly) until effective.
- Withdrawal from drug therapy must be gradual and monitored.

KeyPoints

- Antipsychotics are effective symptomatic treatments for schizophrenia; positive symptoms are more readily treated than negative.
- All drugs are antagonists of dopamine receptors.
- Atypical agents are the drugs of choice.
- Movement disorders are the major side-effects of antipsychotics.

Self-assessment

1. **Fill in the missing words:**
a. Antipsychotic drugs are also known as major tranquillisers and

   _____.
b. All antipsychotics are antagonists of _____ receptors.
c. If two other antipsychotics have proved to be ineffective, _____ should be prescribed.
d. The movement disorder side-effect of _____ can appear months after the start of antipsychotic therapy.

2. **Which of the following statements are true?**
a. Phenothiazines (e.g. chlorpromazine) are highly sedative.
b. Antipsychotics can be used to prevent parkinsonian tremor.
c. Antipsychotics are more effective against the positive than the negative symptoms of schizophrenia.
d. Antipsychotics can be used to treat psychotic dementia in the elderly.

3. **Answer true or false:**
a. Olanzapine is associated with increased risk of stroke in the elderly.
b. Antipsychotics are an effective treatment for akathisia.
c. Emergency intramuscular injection of an antipsychotic should be at a higher dose than when the same drug is given orally.
d. There is no need to change from a typical to an atypical antipsychotic if the patient is responding to treatment.

chapter 23
Parkinson's disease

Parkinson's disease (PD) is a progressive movement disorder of unknown cause related to the degeneration of dopamine-containing neurones in the basal ganglia in the brain. Patients classically present with bradykinesia, rigidity and tremor at rest. PD-like symptoms can be drug-induced (notably by dopamine receptor antagonists such as antipsychotic agents).

The control of voluntary movement is very complex but, simply put, conscious activity in the muscles is driven from the motor cortex via the reticular formation and spinal cord (Figure 23.1). The basal ganglia have a general 'braking' role. For example, in order to sit upright all movements except those reflexes that maintain that posture must be inhibited. Voluntary movement then requires a brake on some of the postural reflexes and release of the brake on muscles required for that movement. The deficits in PD are of two sorts: unwanted movements or difficulty with intended movements.

Figure 23.1 Simplified diagram of the brain areas controlling movement.

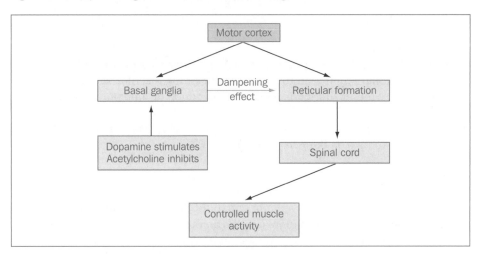

There is no definitive diagnostic test for PD and distinguishing it from similar conditions must be done on the basis of clinical examination and history. Although it is primarily a movement disorder, PD is also associated with dementia, depression, autonomic disturbances and pain. Symptoms are unlikely to appear until a substantial proportion of dopamine-containing neurones in the striatal area of the basal ganglia have died. There are no currently available treatments that halt the progression of the disease.

Antiparkinsonian drugs

There is no single drug of choice for the treatment of early PD. Most patients in the later stages of the disease require levodopa treatment in combination with other anti-PD drugs.

Dopamine receptor agonists
e.g. bromocriptine, cabergoline, pergolide, prampexole, ropinirole, rotigotine, apomorphine

Mechanism of action
- Stimulation of postsynaptic dopamine D_2 receptors in the corpus striatum (part of the basal ganglia).

Adverse effects
- Nausea and vomiting (particularly with apomorphine).
- Ergot-derived drugs (bromocriptine, cabergoline, pergolide) associated with pulmonary, retroperitoneal and pericardial fibrosis; patients should be monitored for breathing difficulties, signs of cardiac failure and abdominal pain.
- Drowsiness with sudden onset of sleep.
- Hallucinations.
- Less commonly, psychosis, pathological gambling, increased libido and hypersexuality.

Clinical context
- Moderate control of symptoms and lack of motor complications (as seen with levodopa) might lead to choice of dopamine receptor agonists as first-line therapy (other first-choice options: levodopa or monoamine oxidase inhibitors).
- The weak dopaminergic agonist amantadine can be used in combination therapy to reduce dyskinesia in advanced PD.

Levodopa
Mechanism of action
- The amino acid levodopa is the precursor of dopamine (and other catecholamines). In PD, it increases the amount of dopamine available for release from surviving dopaminergic neurones in the basal ganglia.
- Given alone, levodopa would be converted to dopamine in the periphery by dopa-decarboxylase, leading to severe nausea and cardiovascular side-effects. Dopamine, unlike levodopa, does not cross the blood–brain barrier.
- Co-administered with the dopa-decarboxylase inhibitors carbidopa or benserazide. These enzyme inhibitors are excluded from the brain, allowing conversion of levodopa to dopamine in the basal ganglia.
- Levodopa/dopa-decarboxylase combination can also be co-administered with the catechol-O-methyltransferase (COMT) inhibitors entacapone or tolcapone to enhance levodopa uptake into the brain.

Adverse effects

- Must be used with caution in patients with severe cardiovascular, pulmonary or psychiatric disease or endocrine disorders affecting autonomic control (e.g. hyperthyroidism).
- Nausea, vomiting and taste disturbances.
- Arrhythmias, postural hypotension, fainting.
- Drowsiness with sudden sleep onset.
- Dementia, psychosis, hallucinations.
- Euphoria and abnormal dreams, but anxiety and depression also possible.
- Dystonia, dyskinesia and chorea; particular problem in younger patients.

Clinical context

- Levodopa is the most effective of the first-choice drug options (only about 10% of patients will not derive significant benefit) but motor complications are problematic.
- The dose should be gradually titrated to minimum effective to help avoid large fluctuations in response (so-called 'on–off' behaviour).
- Responses to levodopa gradually decline, with the period of benefit after each dose becoming shorter.
- Modified-release preparations may be used to reduce motor side-effects in advanced disease.

Monoamine oxidase type B inhibitors

e.g. rasagiline, selegiline

Mechanism of action

- Preservation of releasable dopamine by inhibiting catabolism in surviving dopaminergic neurones in the basal ganglia.
- Selective for type B enzyme so no problematic food interactions (see Chapter 20).

Adverse effects

- Less marked with rasagiline.
- Caution necessary with selegiline in gastric or duodenal ulcer patients, cardiovascular disease (particularly postural hypotension) and psychosis.
- Nausea, gastrointestinal disturbance.
- Postural hypotension, particularly in combination with levodopa.
- Vertigo, abnormal dreams and hallucinations.
- Abrupt withdrawal must be avoided.

Clinical context

- Used alone in the early stages of PD, rasagiline can delay the need to use levodopa.
- Used in combination with levodopa/dopa-decarboxylase inhibitor, rasagiline smooths out 'on–off' and end-of-treatment fluctuations in response.

Antimuscarinic drugs

e.g. benztropine, orphenadrine, procyclidine, trihexyphenidyl (benzhexol)

Mode of action

- Reduce the relatively excessive cholinergic tone in the presence of reduced dopaminergic drive.

Adverse effects

- Caution is required in cardiovascular disease, psychosis and narrow-angle glaucoma.
- Antiparasympathetic nervous system effects: dry mouth, urinary retention, constipation, blurred vision.
- Confusion, memory impairment, hallucinations.
- Reduced skills in motor task performance (e.g. driving).

Clinical context

- Some positive effects on tremor and rigidity but no relief of bradykinesia.
- May be useful in drug-induced parkinsonism but not as effective as dopaminergic drugs, so little place in PD therapy, particularly given their negative effects on cognition.

Catechol-O-methyltransferase inhibitors

e.g. entacapone, tolcapone

- COMT is also involved in the breakdown of dopamine and inhibitors of this enzyme will also increase levels of dopamine and so enhance dopaminergic function.
- Used as adjuncts to levodopa therapy and may smooth out the 'end-of-dose effects'. Levodopa is also a substrate for COMT and its co-administration will prevent peripheral metabolism of L-dopa and so optimise levels of L-dopa for central conversion to dopamine.

KeyPoints

- PD is a progressive neurodegenerative disorder of movement control, involving destruction of dopamine-releasing cells in the basal ganglia.
- Drug therapy controls symptoms but not the disease process (origin unknown).
- Levodopa, in combination with enzyme inhibitors to prevent its peripheral breakdown, is the mainstay of therapy.
- Dopamine receptor agonists and selective monoamine oxidase inhibitors are helpful alone in the early stages of the disease and, later, in combination with levodopa.

Self-assessment

1. Which of the following symptoms are characteristic of PD?
a. bradykinesia
b. muscle tremor

c. depression
d. dementia

2. **Which of the following dopamine receptor agonists used in PD are associated with fibrosis of lung, gut and heart?**
a. bromocriptine
b. pergolide
c. apomorphine
d. amantadine

3. **Which of the following drugs are used to enhance the availability of levodopa for uptake into the brain?**
a. benztropine
b. tolcapone
c. selegiline
d. carbidopa

4. **Which of the following drugs would be first choice in the treatment of early-stage PD?**
a. levodopa
b. rotigotine
c. rasagiline
d. orphenadrine

chapter 24
Analgesics

Analgesics are drugs that reduce the sensation of pain.

- Pain is an unpleasant sensation caused by the processing of sensory information indicating, in a normal physiological context, that damage is occurring in some part of the body. Acute pain is, therefore, a very basic protective mechanism. Chronic, intractable or spontaneous pain serves little useful function.
- Analgesic drugs can operate at the level of pain initiation (e.g. non-steroidal anti-inflammatory drugs (NSAIDs)), transmission of neuronal information (local anaesthetics: LAs) or its processing in the spinal cord and brain (e.g. opioids) (Figure 24.1).

Figure 24.1 Schematic diagram of the main pain pathways. DRG, dorsal root ganglion; NSAIDs, non-steroidal anti-inflammatory drugs.

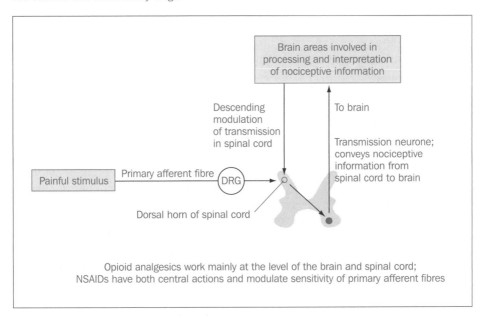

Opioids

e.g. morphine, codeine, diamorphine (heroin), fentanyl, pentazocine, pethidine
- Juice of the opium poppy (*Papaver somniferum*) contains a number of alkaloids, including morphine and codeine.

- Traditionally used for many centuries to produce sleep (as the name suggests), euphoria and analgesia.
- Opiates are compounds structurally related to morphine; opioids are endogenous, plant-derived or synthetic substances that act on the same receptors as morphine and whose effects are blocked by the antagonist naloxone.

Mechanism of action
- Opioids activate μ, κ or δ (MOP, KOP or DOP, G-protein-coupled) receptors causing reduction in cyclic adenosine monophosphate (cAMP), closing of Ca^{2+} ion channels and opening of K^+ channels (see Chapter 3). This hyperpolarises the cells and inhibits neuronal activity in peripheral and central pain circuits.

Adverse effects
- Nausea and vomiting (particularly when first taken)
- Constipation (reduced gastrointestinal motility)
- Respiratory depression (potentially fatal) in overdose
- Drowsiness
- Difficulty with micturition
- Headache
- Dry mouth and sweating
- Reduced libido
- Rashes, urticaria and pruritus (due to release of histamine)
- Mood changes
- Dizziness and postural hypotension.

Clinical context
- Opioids are used to control moderate to severe pain, particularly of visceral origin.
- Despite causing tolerance (requiring increased doses to maintain effective analgesia), regular use may be appropriate for certain types of chronic pain, if used under expert supervision. Induction of psychological dependence is not normally an issue when opioids are used as analgesics.
- In addition to simple pain relief, morphine produces a euphoric, detached state of mind, useful in severe (e.g. postoperative) pain.
- Morphine can be given orally (every 4 h, or less frequently via modified-release preparations), by subcutaneous or intramuscular injection or by slow intravenous injection. Rectal administration is also effective. Opioids can be given epidurally (unlicensed) in postoperative care, but this is associated with multiple side-effects and is scarcely more effective than subcutaneous administration.
- Combination injections of morphine with the antiemetic cyclizine are available.
- Codeine is less effective than morphine and is used for mild/moderate pain, but constipation prevents long-term use. It is used as an antitussive but is only effective at doses causing some degree of respiratory depression.

- Diamorphine and morphine are equally potent analgesics. Diamorphine may cause less nausea and its greater aqueous solubility allows smaller injection volumes, which might be useful in emaciated patients.
- Pethidine is less potent than morphine. It has a rapid onset, brief period of action and is less constipating. Therefore, it is suitable for use in labour.

Other drugs

Non-steroidal anti-inflammatory drugs
e.g. aspirin, ibuprofen, naproxen, indometacin, piroxicam, meloxicam

Mechanism of action
NSAIDs inhibit cyclooxygenases (COX), which metabolise arachidonic acid to prostaglandins and thromboxanes (see Chapter 7). These prostanoids mediate inflammation and potentiate directly painful stimuli. They are also important in temperature control so NSAIDs lower elevated temperature (antipyrexic). The COX-1 enzyme is constitutively active whereas COX-2 is expressed in inflammation.

Adverse effects
- All NSAIDs are associated with serious gastrointestinal side-effects, particularly in the elderly, including pain, nausea, diarrhoea, bleeding and ulceration. Ibuprofen has lowest risk, azapropazone the highest risk. COX-2 inhibitors have much reduced gastrointestinal side-effects but should not be used with existing gastrointestinal symptoms.
- Other adverse effects include hypersensitivity reactions (rashes and bronchospasm: worsening of asthma), headache, dizziness and hearing disturbances (tinnitus). Due to an association with Reye's syndrome (potentially fatal condition affecting brain and liver), aspirin should not be given to children under 16 years of age.
- All NSAIDs are contraindicated in severe heart failure. Selective inhibitors of COX-2 (e.g. celecoxib) are also contraindicated in ischaemic heart disease, cerebrovascular and peripheral arterial disease.

Clinical context
- NSAIDs are useful in acute pain, e.g. headache, transient musculoskeletal, dental, postoperative pain and dysmenorrhoea. Short-term action: aspirin, ibuprofen; longer-acting, naproxen, piroxicam.
- They are used in conjunction with opioids for chronic pain.
- NSAIDs are used long-term for the treatment of rheumatoid and osteoarthritis.

Paracetamol (acetaminophen)
Mechanism of action
- Paracetamol has a similar mechanism of action to NSAIDs but has no anti-inflammatory effects.
- It has been proposed to cause inhibition of a splice variant of COX-1.
- It is not an NSAID.

Adverse effects

- There is much less risk of gastrointestinal side-effects with paracetamol compared with NSAIDs but severe damage to liver in overdose. Only 20–30 tablets taken within 24 h can be fatal; maximum liver damage occurs 3–4 days after ingestion. Acetylcysteine infusion protects the liver if infused within 24 hours.

Clinical context

- As for NSAIDs: short-term action.

Local anaesthetics

e.g. lidocaine, bupivacaine, oxybuprocaine

Applied by injection or surface application to produce local analgesia. Often given with adrenaline to counteract vasodilator effects of LA.

Mechanism of action

- Inhibit action potential conduction in sensory nerves by blocking voltage-operated ('fast') sodium channels.

Adverse effects

- Toxicity arises from systemic overdose; inebriation followed by sedation, twitching, convulsions. Intravenous LA causes convulsions and cardiovascular collapse; care needed to avoid accidental intravascular injection.

Clinical context

- Injections of lidocaine with adrenaline are used for dental analgesia; infiltration anaesthesia, e.g. for minor surgery.
- LA ointments (lidocaine) are used to relieve pain of haemorrhoids and anal fissure.
- Eye drops containing oxybuprocaine, tetracaine or proxymetacaine (less initial stinging; good for children) are used for tonometry or minor ophthalmic surgery.
- Lozenges or ointments containing lidocaine have limited benefit in treating mouth ulcers.
- Topical preparations for treating pruritus (itching) are only marginally effective and can cause sensitisation. Lidocaine patches have some benefit in neuropathic pain (see below).

Antimigraine drugs

Migraine headache can be treated with simple analgesics (paracetamol, ibuprofen) or, if ineffective, with specific antimigraine compound ($5HT_1$ receptor agonists (triptans); almotriptan, eletriptan, sumatriptan, zolmitriptan).

Mechanism of action

- Constriction of dilated meningeal blood vessels by activation of perivascular neurone $5HT_{1B/D}$ receptors and subsequent inhibition of vasodilator neuropeptide release.

Adverse effects

- Triptans are contraindicated if history of stroke, transient ischaemic attacks or peripheral vascular disease.
- Caution is required in coronary artery disease due to risk of vasoconstriction.
- There may be sensations of tingling, heat, tightness of throat or chest, flushing dizziness.

For prophylaxis, pizotifen (a $5HT_2$ receptor antagonist and antihistamine) is used. Other agents which may be used for prevention include sodium valproate, amitriptyline and β-blockers.

Drugs for neuropathic pain treatment

Chronic neuropathic pain can arise from nerve injury or viral infection. It can include spontaneous pain, allodynia (pain due to normally innocuous stimuli, e.g. light brushing, mild cold) or burning pain and is resistant to conventional analgesics.

The antiepileptics gabapentin and pregabalin are effective. The tricyclic antidepressants amitriptyline and nortriptiline are also used (unlicensed). Capsaicin (active ingredient of chilli peppers) is licensed for use, but the initial intense burning sensation it produces makes it unpopular (see Chapter 35). The mechanisms of action of these drugs are uncertain.

Drugs for trigeminal neuralgia

Trigeminal neuralgia is severe (suggested to be the most intense pain experienced in humans), episodic facial pain due to overactivity of trigeminal nerve. The antiepileptic carbamazepine is partially effective, as are the unlicensed oxcarbazepine, gabapentin and lamotrigine. Phenytoin can be given by intravenous infusion in an emergency.

KeyPoints

- Opioid drugs are effective in most severe pain states.
- They are highly toxic (respiratory depression) in overdose and commonly produce constipation and nausea.
- Mild to moderate pain is well controlled by NSAIDs or paracetamol.
- NSAIDs carry a relatively high risk of gastrointestinal side-effects; this is less of a problem for COX-2 inhibitors but these have associated cardiovascular risks.
- LAs are useful for restricted regional analgesia.
- Migraine is most effectively treated with triptans.
- Neuropathic pain is resistant to conventional analgesics but is partially treatable with some antiepileptics.

Self-assessment

1. Which of the following are side-effects of opioids?
a. nausea and vomiting
b. incontinence
c. hypertension
d. pupillary dilatation

2. Which of the following opioids are suitable for maternal use during labour?
a. diamorphine
b. pethidine
c. fentanyl
d. pentazocine

3. Which of the following drugs have anti-inflammatory effects?
a. ibuprofen
b. paracetamol
c. morphine
d. lidocaine

4. Antiepileptic drugs such as carbamazepine are useful for the treatment of which of the following painful conditions?
a. postoperative pain
b. migraine
c. neuropathic pain
d. trigeminal neuralgia

5. NSAIDs are contraindicated in which of the following conditions?
a. pregnancy
b. gastric ulcer
c. heart failure
d. asthma

chapter 25
Drugs of abuse

Drug abuse can be defined as:

> the non-medical self-administration of a substance to produce psychoactive effects, intoxication or altered body image, despite the risks involved (Wills 2005).

In the USA, the *Diagnostic and Statistical Manual of Mental Disorders* (DSM: American Psychiatric Association 1994) defines criteria which specify that an individual must satisfy at least one of the following signs recurrently because of drug abuse:

- failure to fulfil important personal commitments
- abuse of drug in physically hazardous situations
- legal problems related to abuse
- problems in relating to other people due to abuse.

DSM criteria are of limited use: they are rigid, and concentrate on individuals already suffering adverse consequences rather than that person's reasons for drug taking and only apply to regular consumption (ruling out occasional use of cannabis, ecstasy, LSD (lysergic acid diethylamide)?); they would not apply to tobacco.

- Dependence is an inappropriate compulsion to take a drug regularly despite it causing physical, mental/behavioural impairment.
- It sometimes includes the need to avoid withdrawal effects but not all recreational drugs have a significant withdrawal syndrome associated.
- The World Health Organization recommends avoidance of the terms 'psychological' and 'physical dependence' and 'addiction' since they are difficult to distinguish clinically and all drug effects should be biologically explicable.

Common mechanisms

- Most, if not all, drugs of abuse increase neural activity in one of the brain's reward circuits. Drug administration increases the activity of the dopamine-containing neurones extending from the ventral tegmental area to the nucleus accumbens.
- The 'rush' (euphoric effect) with opiates and other drugs is related to their pharmacokinetics; the faster the rate of absorption, the greater the rush. For example, intravenous administration is more effective than oral.

- Short-half-life drugs have greater dependence potential than longer-lasting agents (e.g. heroin more than methadone).

Heroin

- Short-term effects appear soon after a single dose and disappear in a few hours. After an injection, the user reports feeling a surge of euphoria ('rush') accompanied by a warm flushing of the skin, a dry mouth and heavy extremities. Following this initial euphoria, the user goes 'on the nod,' an alternately wakeful and drowsy state. Mental functioning becomes clouded due to the depression of the central nervous system.
- Unwanted effects include respiratory depression (fatal in overdose), constipation.
- Chronic intravenous users may develop collapsed veins, infection of the heart lining and valves, abscesses, cellulitis and liver disease. Pulmonary complications include various types of pneumonia that may result from the poor health condition of the abuser and respiratory depression. Nutritional status tends to be poor. There is a danger of human immunodeficiency virus (HIV) and hepatitis from injecting.
- Withdrawal precipitates craving, restlessness, muscle and bone pain, insomnia, diarrhoea and vomiting, cold flashes with goose bumps ('cold turkey') and kicking movements ('kicking the habit'). Major withdrawal symptoms peak between 48 and 72 hours after the last dose and subside after about a week. Sudden withdrawal by heavily dependent users who are in poor health is occasionally fatal, although heroin withdrawal is considered less dangerous than alcohol or barbiturate withdrawal.

Cocaine

- The powdered, hydrochloride salt form of cocaine can be 'snorted' (inhaled) or dissolved in water and injected. Crack is cocaine that has been converted to the free base. This form of cocaine comes in a rock crystal that can be heated and its vapours smoked. 'Crack' refers to the crackling sound when it is heated.
- Cocaine blocks the reuptake of monoamine neurotransmitters (noradrenaline, dopamine) in the peripheral and central nervous systems.
- Physical effects include constricted blood vessels, dilated pupils and increased temperature, heart rate and blood pressure. The duration of cocaine's immediate euphoric effects, which include hyperstimulation, reduced fatigue and mental alertness, depends on the route of administration. The high from snorting may last 15–30 min, while that from smoking may last 5–10 min.
- There is some tolerance after repeated use but sensitisation is possible. Binges, during which the drug is taken repeatedly and at increasingly high doses, may lead to a state of increasing irritability, restlessness and paranoia and can result in full-blown paranoid psychosis.
- Adverse effects include cardiovascular complications, arrhythmias, heart attack and stroke. Appetite reduction may lead to malnutrition.

Alcohol (ethanol)

- Alcohol is a central nervous system depressant, which has excitatory effects due to disinhibition, i.e. reduced release of inhibitory neurotransmitters such as γ-aminobutyric acid (GABA). For example, reduced GABA release in the ventral tegmentum causes increased dopamine release in the nucleus accumbens, leading to feelings of pleasure.
- Depression of higher brain functions causes hilarity, poor judgement and risk-taking behaviour.
- Large doses irritate stomach (nausea, dyspepsia).
- Alcohol inhibits antidiuretic hormone, causing dehydration (hangover). It is involved in many accidents; alcohol use is a major factor in 25% of males admitted to UK hospitals.
- Long-term drinking leads to: neuropathies (peripheral and central, e.g. Wernicke's encephalopathy – psychosis); myopathies (most seriously, primary cardiomyopathy); hepatotoxicities (cirrhosis most common), haematological disorders.
- Alcoholics are often obese (high calorific intake) but malnourished, particularly vitamin-deficient.
- Suicide is very common in alcoholics: the suicide rate is 80 times higher than in non-alcoholics. Up to 30% of alcoholics die by suicide and up to 50% of all suicide attempts in the UK are made by alcoholics.
- Severe withdrawal syndrome is associated with alcoholism; the most severe form is delirium tremens. Confusion, delusions, tactile and visual hallucinations, convulsions and cardiovascular collapse may ensue (15–50% mortality).

Amphetamines (e.g. dexamphetamine, methamphetamine)

- Increase catecholamine (dopamine, noradrenaline) release from brain and sympathetic nervous system neurones.
- Taken orally or by injection.
- Initially cause increased drive, confidence, sociability, loquacity, physical and (some) mental capacity.
- Later, lethargy and depression.
- Anorexigenic; decreases need for food. Some therapeutic use in this regard.
- High doses increase body temperature, cause hallucinations, paranoia and violence.
- Desire to continue dosing leads to psychological dependence.
- Chronic use can precipitate amphetamine psychosis and possibly neurodegeneration.

Ecstasy (MDMA, 3,4-methylenedioxymethamphetamine)

- Like other amphetamines, MDMA releases monoamine neurotransmitters (5-hydroxytryptamine (5HT), noradrenaline, dopamine).

- It acts as both a stimulant and psychedelic, producing an energising effect as well as distortions in time and perception and enhanced enjoyment from tactile experiences.
- In high doses, MDMA can interfere with temperature regulation. On rare, but unpredictable occasions, this can lead to severe hyperthermia, resulting in liver, kidney, and cardiovascular system failure, and death (danger from drinking too much water).
- Cardiovascular risks are similar to cocaine. In animal studies (adolescents more susceptible) MDMA is neurotoxic.
- About 60% of people who use MDMA report withdrawal symptoms, including fatigue, loss of appetite, depressed feelings and trouble concentrating.

Cannabis

- Preparations of *Cannabis sativa* plant; active compounds called cannabinoids.
- Usually smoked, often with tobacco.
- Main psychoactive component is tetrahydrocannabinol (THC).
- Mimics effects of small endogenous lipid messengers (endocannabinoids, e.g. anandamide); inhibits wide range of neurotransmitter release in the brain and periphery.
- Mild euphoric effect in moderate doses; dysphoric in high doses, particularly in naive users.
- Very low acute toxicity but some concerns about precipitation of psychosis in chronic heavy users; increased recurrence of episodes in patients with schizophrenia.
- Stimulates appetite through actions on feeding centres in the hypothalamus and possibly gut.
- Analgesic and antiemetic.

Benzodiazepines

- Hypnotic/anxiolytic when given orally.
- Produce a rush after injection; liquid-filled temazepam capsules were withdrawn due to injection abuse.
- Very high doses commonly injected (600 mg average compared with 10 mg therapeutic dose).
- Increase the intensity and duration of heroin effects when taken together (although useful for combating opiate withdrawal).
- Large numbers of patients dependent after repeated use; more of a problem with short-half-life agents (e.g. nitrazepam).

LSD

- Some amphetamine-like actions after oral administration.
- Acts as an agonist at $5HT_2$ and dopamine receptors.

Table 25.1 Summary of the different classes of drugs of abuse and their liability to dependence

Drug type	Examples	Dependence liability
Narcotic analgesics	Morphine	Very strong
	Heroin	Very strong
General central nervous system depressants	Ethanol	Strong
	Barbiturates	Strong
	Glutethimide	Moderate
	Anaesthetics	Moderate
Anxiolytic drugs	Benzodiazepines	Moderate
Psychomotor stimulants	Amphetamines	Strong
	Cocaine	Very strong
	Caffeine	Weak
	Nicotine	Very strong
	Ecstasy	Very weak
Psychedelic agents	LSD	Weak or absent
	Mescaline	Weak or absent
	Phencyclidine	Moderate
	Cannabis	Weak
	Ecstasy	Very weak

- Most potent mind-altering substance known (active at 50–200 μg).
- Produces emotional swings, time distortion, visual and auditory hallucinations, synaesthesia (mixing of sensory discrimination; 'see' sounds, 'feel' colours), experience may have mystical overtones.
- 'Bad trips' can involve paranoid psychotic episodes, panic, acute depression, terrifying hallucinations.
- Some evidence for postexposure flashbacks years after use.
- No recognised dependence or withdrawal syndrome.

Treatment

- Goal of treating drug abuse is harm reduction; illicit drug use will always happen. Some drug abusers function appropriately, so why should they stop?
- Minimising dangers to individuals and society is more appropriate than condemning (and banning?).
- Abstinence might be a realistic goal for some but is not the only acceptable outcome.
- Quality-of-life issues and prevention of short- and long-term adverse health consequences are equally important.
- Harm reduction includes needle exchange schemes and provision of health information.
- Psychosocial support from drug abuse agencies is essential.

Pharmacological approaches to treatment
Substitution, e.g. methadone treatment for opiate abuse
- Long-acting synthetic opiate agonist administered orally under supervision for sustained period at dose sufficient to prevent opiate withdrawal.

- Decreases opiate craving without producing rush. Patients stabilised on adequate, sustained dosages of methadone can hold jobs, avoid crime and violence of the street culture; reduces exposure to HIV by stopping injecting.
- Buprenorphine is an opioid receptor partial agonist also used as substitute but can precipitate withdrawal in users dependent on high opiate doses.

Nicotine replacement

- Nicotine-containing gum and sublingual tablets provide slow buccal absorption, avoiding the rewarding bolus obtained by smoking; reduces withdrawal syndrome.
- Clinical trials evidence is mixed: little use in reducing cigarette consumption, craving significantly reduced but 1-year quit rates not greatly affected (17% versus 10% placebo). Nicotine patch results similar: little effect on quit rates irrespective of nicotine dose or patient population. Nicotine nasal sprays also available.
- Buproprion (amfebutamone, Zyban) is registered as an adjunct to smoking cessation treatment. Formerly used as an antidepressant drug (mixed noradrenaline/5HT uptake inhibitor). Significantly reduces craving and extends quit rates. Mechanism of action unknown. Other antidepressants reported to have beneficial effects in alcohol craving but differences between individual agents indicate complex mode of action. Contraindicated in seizure-prone patients.

Antagonist treatments

e.g. naltrexone therapy for opiate addiction

- Long-acting synthetic opiate antagonist; all the effects of self-administered opiates, including euphoria, are completely blocked.
- Few side-effects when taken orally either daily or three times a week for a sustained period of time. Individuals must be medically detoxified and opiate-free for several days before naltrexone can be taken to prevent precipitating opiate abstinence syndrome. Best used in outpatient setting after medical detoxification in a residential setting.
- Theory is that the repeated lack of the desired opiate effects, as well as perceived futility of using the opiate, will break the habit of opiate addiction. Naltrexone itself has no subjective effects or potential for abuse. Patient non-compliance is a major problem.

Alcohol dependence

- Disulfiram is used as an adjunct treatment in withdrawal programmes to prevent further alcohol consumption. It is an attempt at aversion therapy. In the presence of alcohol it leads to the accumulation of acetaldehyde which provokes very unpleasant reactions (headache, nausea, palpitations), possibly resulting in cardiac arrhythmias, hypotension and collapse. Patients must be made aware of dangers of even small amounts of alcohol, e.g. in mouthwashes.

- Acamprosate is used for maintenance of abstinence. It is an *N*-methyl-D-aspartate (NMDA) receptor antagonist; these receptors increase in number in alcoholics and their blockade reduces withdrawal symptoms.
- Sedative hypnotics may be of some use in attenuating withdrawal symptoms. One of these, clomethiazole, also inhibits alcohol dehydrogenase, which slows the rate of alcohol elimination and reduces withdrawal symptoms. Long-acting benzodiazepines (e.g. chlordiazepoxide) are also used but beware of risks of dependence.

References

American Psychiatric Association (1994) *Diagnostic and Statistical Manual of Mental Disorders.* Washington, DC: American Psychiatric Association.

Wills S (2005) *Drugs of Abuse*, 2nd edn. London: Pharmaceutical Press.

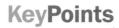

KeyPoints

- All abused drugs have the potential to cause dependence to some extent.
- Most, if not all, drugs of abuse activate dopaminergic reward pathways in the brain.
- Some, but not all, drugs of abuse are associated with withdrawal syndromes.
- The major goal of treatment should be overall harm reduction rather than aiming at complete abstinence.
- Rapidly acting, short-half-life drugs produce a more profound 'high' and greater dependence potential than slowly absorbed, biologically persistent agents.
- Pharmacological treatments can involve substitution with similar, more innocuous drugs or routes of administration, blockade of drug effects, reduction in craving and abstinence syndrome.

Self-assessment

1. Which of the following have a very strong tendency to cause dependence?
   a. cannabis
   b. ecstasy (MDMA)
   c. nicotine
   d. LSD

2. The most intense euphoric effects ('rush') of e.g. cocaine would be produced by administration via which of the following routes?
   a. oral
   b. intravenous
   c. buccal
   d. nasal

3. Which of the following drugs antagonises the effects of heroin?
   a. buprenorphine
   b. methadone
   c. naltrexone
   d. temazepam

4. **Which of the following are used for treating alcoholism?**
a. disulfiram
b. buproprion
c. acamprosate
d. clomethiazole

5. **Withdrawal (abstinence) syndromes are common when regular users of which of the following drugs cease administration?**
a. temazepam
b. cannabis
c. LSD
d. cocaine

chapter 26
General anaesthetics

General anaesthetics (GAs) have made painless surgery possible and have been in use for over 150 years. Despite this, their mechanism of action is uncertain. They should also be distinguished from local anaesthetics (see Chapter 24) which block nervous conduction via inhibition of voltage-operated sodium channels.

General anaesthesia usually involves rapid induction (often with an intravenous agent) followed by maintenance (often with a gaseous agent). The phases of general anaesthesia follow:

- analgesia
- excitation
- surgical anaesthesia
- overdose (e.g. respiratory depression).

In addition to GAs, analgesics (usually opioids; see Chapter 24) and neuromuscular blockers (Chapter 27) are also often used during surgery. Premedications may be used prior to surgery for anxiety/amnesia (e.g. benzodiazepines; see Chapter 19) and to dry up secretions (e.g. antimuscarinic drugs).

Mechanisms of general anaesthetics

- These are incompletely understood.
- Initial theories (Meyer–Overton) related to 'lipid perturbation' in which general anaesthetic properties correlated with lipid solubility. It was thought that the GAs partitioned into the cell membrane and altered cellular function such as ion channel activity. One argument against this as a unitary hypothesis is that some intravenous agents are enantiomer-specific.
- More recent theories suggest that GAs bind to hydrophobic sites in ion channels and alter function. This might include increased activity of inhibitory neurotransmitters such as γ-aminobutyric acid (GABA) and glycine and reduced activity of excitatory neurotransmitters such as N-methyl-D-aspartate (NMDA) and 5-hydroxytryptamine (5HT).
- GAs may also activate certain potassium channels, leading to hyperpolarisation and reduced excitability.
- GAs reduce central nervous system activity and actions on the reticular activating system are thought to lead to unconsciousness or a state of general anaesthesia. Depression of the hippocampus may lead to amnesia.
- The effects of GAs are usually rapidly reversible. In the case of intravenous agents such as thiopental, rapid redistribution (see Chapter 8) leads to reduced plasma concentrations, terminating the anaesthetic effect. Other

agents such as propofol may undergo redistribution and rapid metabolism. Gaseous agents have a short half-life, with the actions being terminated as they are expired from the lungs.

Intravenous agents

- Intravenous agents are usually used for induction. They are usually given at the start of anaesthesia by intravenous injection.
- The effects are rapid, within one 'arm–brain' circulation.
- Thiopental is a barbiturate, and has a well-established action on $GABA_A$-associated chloride channels, leading to increased GABAergic activity. It lacks analgesic activity.
- Propofol may potentiate GABA and glycine-mediated inhibitory effects. It may be given as an infusion for short operations. It is widely used and not associated with a hangover effect.
- Ketamine is an NMDA receptor antagonist. It leads to dissociative anaesthesia with analgesia and amnesia; the patient is unaware of external commands, but may have their eyes open.
- Etomidate enhances GABA activity.

Gaseous agents

- Gaseous agents are usually used for maintenance (but can be used for induction, e.g. sevoflurane, which is less irritating).
- Effectiveness is measured by minimum alveolar concentration (MAC), the concentration in the alveoli which gives anaesthesia (lack of response to surgical stimulation) in 50% of patients. It correlates with lipid solubility of the gas.
- Nitrous oxide may inhibit NMDA receptors. It is a weak GA and may be used with oxygen (50% each) to produce analgesia in obstetrics. Repeated exposure may lead to megaloblastic anaemia.
- Isoflurane, halothane and sevoflurane are halogenated gaseous anaesthetics. Halothane is associated with a risk of hepatotoxicity on repeat exposure.

KeyPoints

- Mechanisms of action are unclear.
- They may involve augmentation of inhibitory systems (e.g. GABA and glycine) and suppression of excitatory systems (e.g. glutamate at NMDA receptors).
- Agents are used for induction and maintenance of anaesthesia.
- Agents are intravenous and gaseous with short half-lives (or redistributed to give a short effective $t_{1/2}$).

Self-assessment

1. **In terms of general anaesthetics, the following are true or false:**
a. There is a single mechanism of action.
b. Barbiturates cause activation of the $GABA_A$-associated chloride channels.
c. General anaesthesia usually involves induction and maintenance.
d. All general anaesthetics are powerful analgesics.
e. MAC correlates with the potency of intravenous general anaesthetics.

chapter 27
Neuromuscular blocking drugs

Drugs that relax skeletal muscle (e.g. abdominal wall) are essential in surgical practice, allowing a low, safe level of anaesthesia to be adopted. They are also used to relax the vocal cords to facilitate intubation. Therapeutically useful drugs work at the neuromuscular junction (NMJ), the synapse between motor nerve and skeletal muscle. The neurotransmitter at the NMJ is acetylcholine, which activates nicotinic acetylcholine receptors (ligand-gated ion channels), leading to muscle fibre depolarisation and contraction.

Non-depolarising neuromuscular blockers

There are two groups:
1. aminosteroids (pancuronium, rocuronium, vecuronium)
2. benzylisoquinoliniums (atracurium, cisatracurium, mivacurium).

Mechanism of action
- These are nicotine receptor antagonists, competing with acetylcholine.

Adverse effects
- Allergic cross-reactivity between different blockers is possible.
- Benzylisoquinolinium drugs cause histamine release, with the possibility of skin flushing, hypotension, bronchospasm and tachycardia.

Clinical context
- These agents are given by intravenous injection; onset is slower than with depolarising neuromuscular blockers.
- The antagonists have different durations of action ranging from short-acting (15–30 min, e.g. mivacurium) to intermediate (30–40 min, e.g. vecuronium) to long-acting (60–120 min, e.g. pancuronium). All durations are dose-dependent. Short to intermediate use is most common.
- Blockers have no anaesthetic or analgesic actions so care must be taken to prevent awareness.
- Breathing muscles are paralysed by blockers so assisted ventilation necessary.
- Paralysis due to all competitive blockers is reversed by increasing competing amounts of acetylcholine at the NMJ using anticholinesterase drugs (neostigmine).

Depolarising neuromuscular blockers

e.g. suxamethonium

Mechanism of action

- Paradoxically, these drugs cause paralysis of skeletal muscle by mimicking the action of acetylcholine at the NMJ, i.e. they are nicotinic receptor agonists.
- Suxamethonium is resistant to hydrolysis by acetylcholine esterase and persistent occupation of the nicotinic receptor leads to inactivation and failure to initiate action potentials.

Adverse effects

- Caution is required if the patient has a history of cardiac, respiratory or neuromuscular disease.
- They are contraindicated if there is a family history of malignant hyperthermia, for major trauma, severe burns and for hyperkalaemia.
- Initial acetylcholine-like action causes skeletal muscle twitches, possibly leading to postoperative muscle pain.
- Suxamethonium is metabolised by pseudocholinesterase; if genetically deficient or if a normal patient is given high or repeated doses, dual block can develop. This has the characteristics of non-depolarising blockade and can be dangerously prolonged. Dual block can be identified by reversal using the short-acting acetylcholine esterase inhibitor edrophonium and fully reversed with neostigmine.

Clinical context

- They have a rapid onset (intravenous injection) and short duration of action (2–6 min, dose-dependent).
- Recovery is spontaneous.
- Acetylcholine esterase inhibitors enhance paralysis.
- They are ideal for very short surgical procedures, e.g. intubation.
- They are applied under anaesthesia to avoid painful muscle twitches.

KeyPoints

- Neuromuscular blockers relax skeletal muscle, facilitating surgical procedures.
- Drugs are either non-depolarising (nicotinic receptor antagonists) or depolarising (nicotinic receptor agonists).
- Depolarising block is very short and recovery is spontaneous; non-depolarising block is more prolonged and reversed by acetylcholine esterase inhibition.

Self-assessment

1. **Which of the following are characteristic of non-depolarising neuromuscular blockade?**
a. very short duration of action
b. assisted ventilation required
c. potentiated by edrophonium
d. associated with histamine release

2. **Which of the following are characteristic of depolarising neuromuscular blockade?**
a. paralysis of long duration
b. paralysis preceded by muscle twitches
c. can develop into dual block
d. reversed by neostigmine

chapter 28
Thyroid disorders

The thyroid gland produces thyroxine (T_4), but also triiodothyronine (T_3), which is the more active hormone; indeed, T_4 may undergo peripheral conversion to T_3. Both of these hormones play important roles in the regulation of cellular metabolism (increasing) and growth, whilst also influencing the activity of the sympathetic nervous system. Overactivity (hyperthyroidism) is managed by reducing the synthesis of thyroid hormones and underactivity (hypothyroidism) is managed by replacing T_4.

Thioamides

Carbimazole and propylthiouracil
- Thioamides decrease the production of thyroid hormones by inhibiting the iodination of thyroglobulin and this occurs via inhibition of thyroperoxidase.
- The thyroid hormones have long plasma half-lives, so it takes several weeks to inhibit their synthesis.
- Thioamides may cause agranulocytosis, leading to leucopenia.

β-blockers

e.g. atenolol, nadolol, propranolol
- These are used to provide symptomatic relief from enhanced sympathetic activity in hyperthyroidism.
- They reduce the actions of catecholamines at β-adrenoceptors, which are augmented in this condition.
- They give symptomatic relief from:
  - tremor
  - anxiety
  - palpitations – diltiazem may control tachycardia in patients who cannot receive a β-blocker.
- Non-selective β-blockers (e.g. propranolol) are required to relieve the tremor.

Levothyroxine

- Restoring thyroid hormone levels is achieved by administration of levothyroxine (T_4).
- T_4 is a prohormone converted in peripheral cells to T_3, which activates intracellular receptors, altering gene transcription.
- The dose required is the one that leads to correct thyroid-stimulating hormone levels.

- Levothyroxine is used with caution in elderly patients, and those with ischaemic heart disease.

KeyPoints

- T_4 is converted to the more active T_3, which acts on nuclear receptors.
- Thioamide inhibits the synthesis of thyroid hormones.
- In hyperthyroidism, β-blockers provide initial symptomatic relief.

Self-assessment

In relation to thyroid disorders, which of the following are true or false?
1. In hyperthyroidism, β-blockers are used to reduce levels of thyroid hormones.
2. Carbimazole is associated with agranulocytosis.
3. There is increased sympathetic activity in hyperthyroidism.
4. Thioamides cause a rapid normalisation of thyroid levels.
5. Levothyroxine acts on a G-protein-coupled transmembranous receptor.

chapter 29
Diabetes mellitus

Type 1 diabetes

- Type 1 diabetes is generally associated with onset at a young age (<40 years old).
- It may be caused by destruction of pancreatic β-cells following certain viral infections or due to an autoimmune process.
- It is characterised by an inability of the β-cells to produce insulin and is fatal if not treated.

Insulin
- Replace endogenous insulin to return blood glucose to normal and prevent diabetic complications.
- Insulin binds to its transmembranous receptor, leading to activation of tyrosine kinase which causes autophosphorylation and phosphorylation of other proteins (see Chapter 2).
- Insulin receptor activation leads to cellular uptake of glucose via Glut-4 transporter, increased glycogen synthesis, decreased gluconeogenesis and effects on cell growth.
- Insulin lowers blood glucose.
- Human insulin analogues: modified insulin peptides (insulin lispro and insulin aspart) have a rapid onset but short duration of action.
- Short-acting insulins have relatively short-lived effects of 6–8 h, with peak effects at 2–5 h. These are given approximately 15–30 min before meals.
- Intermediate- and long-acting insulins: combination of insulin with protamine gives rise to intermediate-acting insulin (isophane insulin), binding to zinc gives intermediate to long-acting insulin and combination with protamine plus zinc gives long-acting insulin.

Type 2 diabetes

- Type 2 diabetes is associated with increased insulin resistance – tissues become less responsive to insulin, which leads to increased blood glucose levels.
- β-cells still produce insulin but there may be loss of cells or reduced glucose sensitivity.
- Associated diseases:
  - obesity
  - hypertension
  - hyperlipidaemia.
- Generally presents after the age of 40 years.

Diet

- Initially manage by dietary modification, weight loss and increased exercise.
- If this fails to control the condition then antidiabetic drugs are used.

Biguanides

Metformin
- Its action is unclear, but may involve activation of adenosine monophosphate (AMP)-activated protein kinase.
- Actions may include:
  - increased glucose uptake into muscle
  - reduced absorption of glucose from the gastrointestinal tract
  - reduced output of glucose from the liver.
- It is the drug of choice for most (especially obese) patients.
- Metformin does not cause hypoglycaemia.
- It should not be used in renal impairment.

Sulphonylureas

e.g. glibenclamide, gliclazide, tolbutamide

Mechanism of action
- Sulphonyulureas increase insulin secretion.
- They inhibit adenosine triphosphate (ATP)-sensitive potassium (K_{ATP}) channels (see Chapter 4).
- Glucose leads to ATP production, which inhibits these channels, leading to cellular depolarisation, which results in calcium influx and insulin secretion.
- When glucose is low, ATP levels fall and adenosine diphosphate (ADP) rises, channels open, with membrane hyperpolarisation, and this decreases insulin release.
- Sulphonylureas bind to a receptor associated with these channels, resulting in channel closure, which leads to insulin release.

Adverse effects
- Insulin secretion is associated with weight gain and hypoglycaemia.

Meglitinide analogues

e.g. nateglinide, repaglinide
- These also act on β-cells but interact with the sulphonylurea receptor in a slightly different manner than sulphonylureas to cause closure of the K_{ATP}-channels, leading to depolarisation and insulin release.
- They have a rapid rate of onset and are given at meal times to stimulate postprandial insulin secretion, which is relatively short-lived.

- Their effects may be enhanced by the patient having a meal and they are referred to as prandial glucose regulators (PGRs).

Thiazolidinediones ('glitazones')

e.g. pioglitazone, rosiglitazone
- Thiazolidinediones activate nuclear peroxisome proliferator-activated receptor-γ (PPAR-γ), which alters gene expression and results in insulin-like effects (see Chapter 2).
- They are 'insulin sensitisers' which work by enhancing glucose utilisation in tissues, and so reduce insulin resistance.
- Effects include:
  - reduced hepatic glucose output
  - increased glucose transporters (GLUT) in skeletal muscle with increased peripheral glucose utilisation
  - increased fatty acid uptake into adipose cells
  - anti-inflammatory.

Glucosidase inhibitors

Acarbose
- Acarbose competitively inhibits the α-glucosidases which metabolise oligosaccharides to monosaccharides in the small intestine brush border epithelium.
- It reduces the production of glucose in the gastrointestinal tract, thereby preventing sharp rises in blood glucose after a meal.
- The subsequent increased presence of carbohydrates in the gastrointestinal tract may lead to flatulence and osmotic diarrhoea as side-effects.

Modulation of incretins

Exenatide, sitagliptin
- Incretins are endogenous hormones which regulate the endocrine pancreas.
- Exenatide is an incretin mimetic which acts on β-cells of the islets of Langerhans to stimulate the release of insulin and also reduces glucagon release.
- Sitagliptin is a dipeptidyl peptidase-4 inhibitor which inhibits the breakdown of incretins and so enhances their action, promoting insulin secretion and suppressing glucagon release.

KeyPoints

- Type 1 diabetes requires insulin.
- Insulin receptors have tyrosine kinase activity.
- Type 2 diabetes is managed by diet and antidiabetic drugs.
- Metformin may activate AMP-activated protein kinase.
- Sulphonylureas inhibit ATP-sensitive potassium channels and stimulate insulin secretion.
- Thiazolidinediones activate nuclear PPAR-γ and sensitise towards insulin.

Self-assessment

1. **Which of the following stimulate insulin secretion from β-cells of the islets of Langerhans?**
a. metformin
b. hyperpolarisation
c. glucose via ATP
d. sulphonylureas
e. exenatide

2. **Which of the following drugs are likely to cause hypoglycaemia?**
a. insulin
b. metformin
c. sulphonylureas
d. acarbose

3. **Match the following drugs to modes of action: insulin, metformin, sulphonylureas, thiazolidinediones:**
a. PPAR-γ activation
b. intrinsic tyrosine kinase activation
c. stimulation of ATP-sensitive potassium channels
d. AMP kinase activation
e. inhibition of ATP-sensitive potassium channels

chapter 30
Antibacterial agents

Antibacterial agents revolutionised medicine in the 20th century by enabling many infections to be managed. 'Antibacterial agents' is the general term and this includes antibiotics, which are chemicals derived from biological organisms which fight infection. For example, the penicillins are derived from moulds and are used to fight bacterial infections.

- Antibacterial agents result in the killing of bacteria (bactericidal) or suppress their growth (bacteriostatic).
- Antibacterial agents work on the principle of selective toxicity, where they target bacterial processes (e.g. cell wall synthesis, protein synthesis) but leave the eukaryotic cells largely unaffected.
- Broad-spectrum agents are effective against a range of organisms.
- Widespread use of antibiotics has resulted in resistance, leading to 'superbugs' which are unaffected by many antibacterials.
- Broad-spectrum antibiotics are associated with diarrhoea as they may disturb the balance of bacterial flora in the gastrointestinal tract.

Penicillins

e.g. amoxicillin, ampicillin, benzylpenicillin (penicillin G), flucloxacillin, phenoxymethylpenicillin (penicillin V)
- β-lactam antibiotics.
- Penicillins target bacterial cell wall synthesis, by binding irreversibly to a transpeptidase, which cross-links peptidoglycans in the bacterial cell wall, and so are only effective against dividing organisms.
- Penicillins are bactericidal, causing lysis of the bacteria.
- Some penicillins are inactivated by β-lactamases secreted by resistant bacteria. Clavulanic acid is included with some agents (e.g. amoxicillin) to inhibit the β-lactamases. Other pencillins (e.g. flucloxacillin) are resistant to β-lactamases.
- Penicillins are immunogenic and some patients develop allergic reactions on repeat exposure.

Cephalosporins

e.g. cefaclor, cefalexin, cefotaxime, cefuroxime
- β-lactam antibiotics.
- Cephalosporins act in a similar way to penicillins.
- They show cross-reactivity with penicillins and approximately 0.5–6.5% of penicillin-allergic patients will also be allergic to cephalosporins.

Glycopeptides

e.g. teicoplanin, vancomycin
- These also inhibit bacterial cell wall synthesis by inhibiting the growth of the peptidoglycan chain.
- They are often used to manage severe infections due to 'superbugs', such as meticillin-resistant *Staphylococcus aureus* (MRSA).
- They are largely bacteriostatic.

Tetracyclines

e.g. doxycycline, tetracycline
- Tetracyclines inhibit protein synthesis, by binding to the 30S subunit of the bacterial ribosome and preventing tRNA from binding at the acceptor (A) site.
- They are bacteriostatic.
- Their use has decreased due to resistance.

Macrolides

e.g. clarithromycin, erythromycin
- Macrolides prevent the translocation of the 50S subunit of the bacterial ribosome along the mRNA and so prevent protein synthesis, resulting in bacteriostatic action.
- Erythromycin is often used as an alternative to penicillin in patients with a penicillin allergy.
- Macrolides are cytochrome P450 inhibitors and associated with a range of drug interactions (increase concentrations of interacting drugs).
- Erythromycin stimulates gastrointestinal motility (via motilin receptors) and is associated with nausea.

Clindamycin

- Clindamycin inhibits protein synthesis by a similar mechanism to the macrolide antibiotics.

Chloramphenicol

- Chloramphenicol inhibits protein synthesis by binding to the 50S subunit of the bacterial ribosome and inhibiting the formation of peptide bonds (transpeptidation).
- Its systemic use is associated with a risk of aplastic anaemia and so is reserved for life-threatening infections.
- Topical chloramphenicol is available as an over-the-counter medicine for conjunctivitis and is not associated with aplastic anaemia.

Aminoglycosides

e.g. gentamicin, neomycin, tobramycin

- Aminoglycosides bind irreversibly to the 30S subunit of bacterial ribosomes, leading to misreading of mRNA and inhibition of protein synthesis.
- They enter the bacterial cells via an energy-dependent active transport process and are therefore less effective against anaerobes.
- They are bactericidal.
- Their use is complicated by toxicity, leading to ototoxicity and nephrotoxicity.

Quinolones

e.g. ciprofloxacin, norfloxacin, ofloxacin

- These are inhibitors of bacterial DNA gyrase and topoisomerase IV.
- In Gram-negative bacteria, DNA gyrase is inhibited and quinolones inhibit the supercoiling of the bacterial DNA, which is essential for DNA repair and replication.
- In Gram-positive bacteria, topoisomerase IV is the target and quinolones interfere with the separation of DNA strands on replication.

Sulphonamides and trimethoprim

- Sulphonamides are analogues of *p*-aminobenzoic acid (PABA) and inhibit the growth of bacteria by competitively inhibiting the enzyme dihydropteroate synthase, involved in the synthesis of folate from PABA.
- The availability of DNA and RNA precursors is, therefore, reduced.
- They are bacteriostatic.
- Human metabolism is not affected as folate is obtained from the diet.
- Trimethoprim is structurally related to folate, thereby acting as a folate antagonist and inhibiting the bacterial dihydrofolate reductase, which converts folate to tetrahydrofolate. Trimethoprim is less potent against the human form of the enzyme.
- Trimethoprim is used in urinary tract and chest infections.
- Sulphamethoxazole is combined with trimethoprim in co-trimoxazole.

Metronidazole

- This is a pro-drug which is activated by anaerobic bacteria to products which damage the helical structure of DNA.
- It is used against anaerobic bacteria and protozoa.
- It leads to a disulfiram reaction with alcohol.

Antituberculous drugs

These drugs are used in combination to eradicate tuberculosis infections due to mycobacteria. Treatment is required for 6–9 months to cure the infection.

Isoniazid

- Isoniazid inhibits synthesis of mycolic acid present in mycobacteria cell walls.
- It possesses selective bacteriostatic activity against mycobacteria species with some bactericidal activity against the actively dividing mycobacteria.

Rifampicin

- Rifampicin binds to and inhibits DNA-dependent RNA polymerase in prokaryotic cells but not eukaryotic cells.
- It is also active against some Gram-positive and Gram-negative species.
- It is an important inducer of drug metabolism via induction of cytochrome P450 (decreases the concentrations of interacting drugs).

Ethambutol

- Ethambutol inhibits the growth of mycobacteria through inhibition of arabinosyl transferases involved in cell wall synthesis.
- Resistance is a problem.

Pyrazinamide

- This agent becomes tuberculostatic at acidic pH.
- It is effective against intracellular mycobacteria found in macrophages following phagocytosis.
- Pyrazinamide is most effective against rapidly dividing intracellular organisms and is most effective in the first 2 months.

KeyPoints

- Bacterial cell wall synthesis is the target for penicillins, cephalosporins and glycopeptides.
- Bacterial protein synthesis and the bacterial ribosomal subunits are the targets for tetracyclines, macrolides, clindamycin, chloramphenicol and aminoglycosides.
- Quinolones inhibit the bacterial DNA gyrase.
- Sulphonamides and trimethoprim interfere with the bacterial synthesis/metabolism of folates, required for DNA and RNA.
- Antibacterial agents are bactericidal or bacteriostatic.

Self-assessment

1. Which of the following antibacterial agents interfere with bacterial wall synthesis?
a. erythromycin
b. amoxicillin
c. chloramphenicol
d. vancomycin
e. ciprofloxacin

2. Pair up the following antibacterial agents with appropriate complications of their usage:

Antibacterial agent

a. erythromycin
b. amoxicillin
c. chloramphenicol (oral)
d. rifampicin
e. gentamicin

Complication

1. ototoxicity
2. aplastic anaemia
3. drug interactions due to enzyme induction
4. drug interactions due to enzyme inhibition
5. destruction by β-lactamase

chapter 31
Non-bacterial infections: antiviral, antifungal and antiparasitic drugs

Antiviral drugs

In drug therapy of viral infections it has proven difficult to exploit differences between viral processes and the host cells. Antiviral drugs tend to suppress viral activity but do not eradicate infections. For example, in herpes infections, antivirals have to be given at the start of an attack to limit the infection.

Aciclovir
- Aciclovir is a nucleoside analogue which undergoes phosphorylation to its monophosphate in virus-infected cells via viral thymidine kinase.
- The monophosphate is then converted to the triphosphate which inhibits the viral DNA polymerase and so prevents viral DNA synthesis and replication.
- Aciclovir triphosphate may also be incorporated in viral DNA and cause chain termination.
- It is used in herpes infections and some cases of chickenpox (varicella), e.g. in severely affected adults.

Ganciclovir
- Ganciclovir is a guanine analogue which is phosphorylated in herpes-infected cell to the monophosphate.
- The triphosphate inhibits the herpes and cytomegalovirus DNA polymerase to inhibit DNA synthesis.

Viral neuramidase inhibitors
e.g. zanamivir, oseltamivir
- These inhibit the viral neuramidases and prevent the entry and release of viral particles from host cells.
- These drugs are effective against influenza A and B.

Anti-HIV drugs
These have substantially improved the outlook for patients infected with human immunodeficiency virus (HIV) and may keep the infection in check for a

substantial time. There are four main classes of antiretroviral drugs and they are used in combination (usually three) to attack different stages of the viral cycle.

Nucleoside reverse transcriptase inhibitors

e.g. didanosine, zidovudine (AZT)

- Phosphorylated by host cells to 5'-triphosphates, which are incorporated into viral DNA by viral reverse transcriptase.
- Leads to chain termination.

Non-nucleoside reverse transcriptase inhibitors

e.g. efavirenz

- Bind to and inactivate viral reverse transcriptase.

Protease inhibitors

e.g. indinavir

- Inhibit the viral protease which is involved in maturation of viral particles and is essential for infectivity.

Fusion inhibitors

e.g. enfuvirtide

- Inhibit the interaction of a viral glycoprotein with the CD4 cell membrane and so prevent virus entering host cell.
- Used when there is resistance to other drugs.

Antifungal agents

Fungal infections may be superficial (skin, nails) or more deeply seated. They include tinea (e.g. athlete's foot) and candidiasis (e.g. thrush) infections. Drugs are given either topically or orally.

Imidazoles (e.g. clotrimazole, miconazole) and triazoles (e.g. itraconazole, fluconazole).

- Imidazoles and triazoles inhibit a cytochrome P450-dependent demethylase which converts lanosterol to ergosterol, a fungal membrane lipid. This results in the accumulation of lanosterol which disrupts the membrane phospholipids.
- Imidazoles and triazoles are fungistatic and so must be used after healing to prevent a relapse.
- Imidazoles and triazoles are widely used in superficial skin infections and are effective against both tinea and candidial infections.
- Oral administration or systemic absorption risks drug interactions via inhibition of cytochrome P450.

Polyenes

e.g. amphotericin B, nystatin

- Polyenes bind to fungal ergosterol in the cell membrane and disrupt the cells by forming pores.
- They are effective in candidiasis but not tinea.

Allylamines
Terbinafine
- Terbinafine inhibits the conversion of squalene to lanosterol by squalene epoxidase, with the accumulation of squalene causing cell death.
- Fungicidal and shorter treatment courses are required.

Griseofulvin
- Griseofulvin binds fungal tubulin and disrupts mitotic spindles involved in cell division.
- It is suitable for tinea infections but not candidiasis, as it is ineffective against the yeast.

Antimalarial agents

These are used as preventive medicines to prevent infection with mosquito-borne malarial protozoal parasites (*Plasmodium*) or to fight infection. Resistance is a problem and the choice of agent is determined by region visited.

4-aminoquinolones (chloroquine)
- Chloroquine binds to haemoglobin breakdown products and becomes concentrated in erythrocytes.
- It inhibits the parasitic haem polymerase used to metabolise haem.
- Haem accumulates and this is toxic to the parasite.
- It is only effective against erythrocytic forms of infection.
- It is used for prophylaxis and treatment.

Quinolone methanols (quinine, mefloquine)
- Similar action to chloroquine.
- Mefloquine is associated with causing depression.
- Mefloquine is mostly used for prophylaxis and quinine for treatment.

Folate antagonists (proguanil, pyrimethamine)
- Folate antagonists inhibit parasitic dihydrofolate reductase and limit availability of folate.
- They have a similar action to trimethoprim (see Chapter 30).
- Proguanil is used for prophylaxis.
- Pyrimethamine is given with a sulphonamide-like drug.

8-aminoquinolones (primaquine)
- Primaquine possibly inhibits parasitic mitochondrial function during infection of liver.
- Metabolites may bind to parasitic DNA.
- It is used for treatment.

Doxycycline
This antibacterial agent may be used for prophylaxis if antimalarials are contraindicated or there is resistance.

Artemether with lumefantrine

- New.
- Inhibits the parasitic conversion of toxic haem to haemozoin in erythrocytes during active infection.
- Used for treatment.

Anthelmintics

e.g. mebendazole, piperazine

- Anthelmintics are used to manage parasitic threadworm and roundworm infections.
- Piperazine activates GABA-associated chloride channels in the worms, causing muscular relaxation and their expulsion from the gut.
- Mebendazole inhibits microtubular function in worms.

Insecticides

Organophosphorus compounds

e.g. malathion, carbaryl

- These are used to manage lice.
- They inhibit acetylcholinesterase and so breakdown of acetylcholine in the louse is blocked, leading to paralysis and death.

Permethrin

- Permethrin activates sodium channels in the louse, leading to paralysis.

KeyPoints

- Antiviral therapy is limited regarding selectivity, e.g. aciclovir is activated in infected cells and leads to inhibition of viral DNA polymerase.
- Anti-HIV therapy is used in combination to attack different stages of the viral cycle.
- Antifungal therapy largely focuses on membrane biochemistry.
- Imidazoles and azoles are important cytochrome P450 inhibitors and this may lead to drug interactions.
- Antimalarial drugs are used for prophylaxis or treatment.

Self-assessment

Match up the following drugs (or classes of drugs) with mechanisms and action and uses:

Drug	Mechanism of action	Use
1. aciclovir	a. folate antagonist	f. antimalarial
2. zanamivir	b. inhibits conversion of lanosterol to ergosterol	g. herpes
3. zidovudine	c. neuramidase inhibitor	h. anti-HIV
4. clotrimazole	d. inhibits viral DNA polymerase	i. influenza
5. proguanil	e. nucleoside reverse transcriptase inhibitor	j. antifungal

chapter 32
Anticancer drugs

Cancer is a major killer in the western world; in the UK, approximately 25% of registered deaths cite cancer as a significant factor. The treatment of cancer is complex and dependent on the type of cancer concerned; however, some principles are common to all cancers.

- Cancer is a malignant neoplasm, in which cells undergo:
  - unchecked cellular proliferation (expand in numbers without limit)
  - tissue invasion (intrude upon and destroy neighbouring normal cells)
  - metastasis (spread to other tissues in the body).
- Cancer kills because of:
  - organ failure
  - destruction/compression of vital structures.
- To give relief (palliation), induce remission or cure, treatment includes:
  - surgery
  - radiotherapy
  - chemotherapy
  - combinations thereof.

Cancer initiation and prevention

Carcinogenesis is the transformation of a normal cell into one that is neoplastic.

- The transformation of a normal cell into a neoplastic cell typically involves mutation of either tumour promoter or tumour suppressor genes.
- With regard to tumour promoters:
  - they enhance proliferation (mitogens) or prevent cell death (antiapoptotic)
  - oncogenes are genes which are involved in the initiation and development of cancer
  - proto-oncogenes are normal genes, usually associated with cell growth and/or division, which become oncogenic after mutation or overexpression.
- Tumour suppressors:
  - inhibit cell cycle progression
  - often function as 'off-switches' in signal transduction pathways.
- Cells in which a mutation has arisen are more inclined to subsequent mutations.
- Most cancerous cells start as clones (exact copies of the first mutated cell).
- Subsequently, cells diversify with repeated division:
  - repair mechanisms have insufficient time to correct DNA damage.

The causes of cancer have been ascribed to a wide variety of stimuli, which can be divided into the following broad groups:

- Chemical carcinogens, which include tobacco smoke and asbestos, as well as less obviously irritant chemicals, such as alcohol and saturated fats. Chemical carcinogens may give rise directly to mutations in cellular DNA or impede the ability of cells to self-repair, thereby leading to daughter cells with an increased number of mutations. Typically, chemical carcinogens act in a tissue-specific manner (usually influenced by the method of contact), so that tobacco smoking gives rise to cancers of the lungs or mouth, while increased saturated fat intake is associated with cancers of the lower bowel.
  - Polycyclic aromatic hydrocarbons, such as anthracene and pyrene, intercalate between basepairs in DNA to cause frameshift mutations.
  - Alkylating agents, such as ethylnitrosourea, can irreversibly bind to DNA, giving rise to point mutations.
- Ionising radiation:
  - Increased exposure to the ultraviolet rays in sunlight is linked with cancer, particularly melanoma of the skin.
- Pathogens, particularly viruses, can give rise to cancers.

Infectious diseases

Some cancers are triggered by pathogens. Viruses, such as human papillomavirus (HPV), hepatitis B and C and Epstein–Barr virus (EBV), account for about 15% of human cancers, probably the second most important risk factor after tobacco. The viral DNA either encodes an oncogene which inserts into the host DNA or else the viral DNA inserts in close proximity to a host proto-oncogene, resulting in overexpression of the proto-oncogene and unchecked cell division.

- Acutely transforming viruses:
  - encode an oncogene which inserts into the host DNA
  - initiate cancer formation with short latency.
- With regard to slowly transforming viruses:
  - they insert DNA in close proximity to a host proto-oncogene, resulting in overexpression of the proto-oncogene and unchecked cell division
  - because the site of insertion is random, the chance of insertion near any proto-oncogene is low
  - they cause tumours much longer after infection.

Vaccines to treat viral-induced cancers are currently limited to hepatitis B and HPV, the latter targeted at pubescent and prepubescent females, with a view to immunise those individuals prior to sexual experience. DNA vaccines are in development.

A major risk factor for stomach cancer is the presence of the pathogen *Helicobacter pylori* in the stomach (see Chapter 9).

Heredity

- The majority of cancers are not inherited.
- However, some tumour suppressor alleles are associated with cancers:
  - *BRCA1* and *BRCA2* genes are involved in DNA repair.

Particular variants increase the risk of breast and ovarian cancers.
- The *APC* gene has a role in cell migration, adhesion, chromosome segregation, spindle assembly and apoptosis.

Particular variants are associated with familial adenomatous polyposis and colon cancers.

Anticancer drugs

- Anticancer drugs are highly successful in some high-mortality cancers, such as:
  - childhood acute lymphoblastic leukaemia
  - testicular cancer
  - Hodgkin's lymphoma
- Some cancers, however, are almost entirely refractory to chemotherapy.
- In general, anticancer drugs are more toxic than other groups of drugs, and so careful risk–benefit analysis must be conducted.

In general, anticancer drugs can be divided into two types: drugs interfering with DNA and its replication and drugs described as 'targeted' therapy.
- In many cases, combination therapy means that a synergistic enhancement of clinical efficacy can be achieved, provided:
  - each drug is individually effective
  - drugs have independent mechanisms
  - drugs show minimal cross-resistance
  - drugs have distinct toxic effects.

Drugs interfering with DNA and its replication

Antimetabolites
- Folic acid inhibitors:
  - Methotrexate inhibits dihydrofolate reductase to decrease thymidylate, purine nucleotide, amino acid levels.
- Purines:
  - Mercaptopurine and thioguanine are activated by hypoxanthine phosphoribosyltransferase to toxic metabolites.
- Pyrimidines:
  - Fluorouracil, cytarabine, gemcitabine.

DNA-damaging drugs

These include alkylating agents, such as cyclophosphamide and cisplatin, and the anthracene antibiotics.
- Cyclophosphamide:
  - prodrug activated in the liver to aldophosphamide then to phosphoramide nitrogen mustard

- aldehyde dehydrogenase diverts aldophosphamide to carboxyphosphamide and so cyclophosphamide is more effective in tissues with a lower aldehyde dehydrogenase activity.
- Cisplatin:
  - pro-drug of inorganic *cis*-platinum
  - *trans*-platinum much less effective.
- Anthracene antibiotics, such as doxorubicin and daunorubicin, interfere with nucleotide synthesis by:
  - intercalating between DNA strands
  - inhibiting topoisomerase
  - generating iron-dependent free radicals.

Topoisomerase inhibitors
- Topoisomerases are a group of enzymes which 'relax' supercoiled DNA, an essential step in DNA replication:
  - inhibited by etoposide, a podophyllotoxin.

Microtubule inhibitors
- Block the formation of the mitotic spindle.
- Include drugs derived from natural products such as the vinca alkaloids, vincristine and vinblastine, as well as paclitaxel and docetaxel.

Targeted therapies

Targeted therapies for cancer include agents targeting hormones, including conventional antagonists and enzyme inhibitors, as well as monoclonal antibodies. A second route for targeted therapy is through the use of inhibitors of intracellular signalling cascades.

Antihormonal agents
- Glucocorticoid agonists, e.g. prednisolone, which elicit immunosuppression, via agonist actions at glucocorticoid receptors.
- Gonadal hormone antagonists:
  - e.g. tamoxifen, which inhibits proliferation of particular breast cancers by antagonising oestrogen receptors
  - e.g. flutamide, which inhibits the progression of some prostate cancers by antagonising androgen receptors.
- Enzyme inhibitors:
  - e.g. anastrozole, which reduces proliferation of some breast cancers by inhibiting aromatase activity and the production of oestrogens
  - e.g. finasteride, which reduces the proliferation rate of cells in benign prostatic hyperplasia, by inhibiting the production of dihydrotestosterone by 5α-reductase.
- Gonadotrophin-releasing hormone (GnRH) analogues (see Chapter 35):
  - e.g. goserelin used in the treatment of particular breast and prostate cancers, acting to reduce the secretion of gonadal hormones.

Examples of monoclonal antibodies

- Bevacizumab: anti-VEGF (vascular endothelial growth factor) to reduce angiogenesis and hence metastasis in advanced colon or breast cancer as an adjuvant
- Rituximab: anti-CD20, targeting leukocytes in non-Hodgkin's lymphoma
- Trastuzumab: ErbB2 (Her-2) inhibitor to reduce epidermal growth factor (EGF) receptor signalling and hence proliferation of particular breast cancers.

Examples of drugs targeting signalling cascades

- Imatinib:
  - targets PDGF receptor signalling by inhibiting tyrosine kinase activities
  - in chronic myeloid leukaemia, a translocation between chromosomes 9 and 22, known as the Philadelphia chromosome, results in fusion of two proteins to form BCR-Abl, a constitutively active tyrosine kinase, which may be inhibited by imatinib with relative selectivity.
- Erlotinib and gefitinib:
  - EGF receptor tyrosine kinase inhibitors used to treat lung and pancreatic cancers.

Drug resistance

- A major issue in cancer therapy.
- Increased DNA repair, particularly important for alkylating agents and cisplatin.
- Formation of trapping agents/chelators: increased glutathione levels negate the action of cisplatin and the anthracyclines.
- Enzyme plasticity: changes in substrate affinity and enzyme expression levels.
- Decreased conversion of prodrugs: particularly relevant for nucleoside antimetabolites (e.g. mercaptopurine, fluorouracil).
- Increased metabolism of drugs: particularly relevant for nucleoside antimetabolites (e.g. mercaptopurine, fluorouracil).
- Increased extrusion of drugs: increased expression of the adenosine triphosphate (ATP)-binding cassette transporter ABCA2 (multidrug resistance protein 1, P-glycoprotein) is responsible for reducing intracellular concentrations of anticancer drugs.

Side-effects of anticancer drugs and rescue therapy

- Extended administration of the anticancer drugs which interfere with DNA and target fast-growing cells can also lead to toxic effects in non-cancerous tissues (e.g. gastrointestinal tract and bone marrow), which also turn over rapidly.
- A cyclical treatment regimen is often employed to allow non-target tissues to recover between bouts of chemotherapy.

- Myelosuppression (suppression of bone marrow activity) is a major adverse effect for most anticancer drugs and leads to anaemia, decreased resistance to infection and increasing bleeding due to reduced platelet counts.
- Patients are therefore immunocompromised and may require antibiotics and antifungal agents. The recovery of white blood cell counts may be enhanced by giving colony-stimulating factors (CSFs) to stimulate leukocyte production.
- Treatment with methotrexate depletes levels of folic acid, so folinic acid supplementation is used as a replacement.
- Cyclophosphamide is hydrolysed to acrolein, a reactive aldehyde, which may be scavenged by mercaptoethanesulphonate (mesna).
- DNA-damaging effects of doxorubicin treatment are partly mediated through iron-catalysed free radical generation, so dexrazoxane is administered to mop up iron.
- Many anticancer agents cause nausea and vomiting.

Palliative care and additional symptom control

Alongside the primary symptoms of the cancer, a number of additional symptoms may present, including pain, nausea, vomiting and diarrhoea. Pain medication often involves the use of opioids, such as diamorphine and oxycodone, while antiemetics, such as ondansetron, granisetron and aprepitant allow stronger medication to be employed.

KeyPoints

- Anticancer drugs may be divided into those interfering with DNA and targeted therapies.
- Anticancer drugs are generally more toxic than most other sorts of drugs.
- Anticancer drugs that interfere with DNA also target rapidly dividing cells in the gastrointestinal tract and bone marrow, leading to additional complications.

Self-assessment

Fill in the gaps in the following sentences:

1. Particular alleles of the *BRCA1* gene predispose to _____ cancer.
2. _____ infection is associated with an elevated risk of gastric cancer.
3. Methotrexate inhibits the enzyme _____.
4. Cyclophosphamide action can be diverted in tissues expressing high activities of the enzyme _____.
5. Etoposide, a podophyllotoxin, inhibits activity of the enzyme _____.
6. Vincristine inhibits _____ function.
7. Tamoxifen is used to treat breast cancers by blocking _____ receptors.
8. _____ is a monoclonal antibody which targets one of the subunits of the EGF receptor in the treatment of some breast cancers.
9. The Philadelphia chromosome is a translocation of chromosomes, and is associated with _____ leukaemia.
10. A major cause of drug resistance is an increased expression of the _____ transporter.

chapter 33
Steroids

Steroids are a series of structurally related endogenous compounds derived from cholesterol and are mainly generated in the adrenal cortex and gonads, although other tissues are sites of synthesis, e.g. neurosteroids in the central nervous system. They are associated with long-term responses, including cell growth and maturation, involving processes such as sexual characteristics and bone density, as well as regulating pathological processes like hormonal dysfunction and cancer.

Steroid nomenclature

The common structure of steroid hormones is composed of at least 20 carbon atoms arranged into four rings, labelled A–D (Figure 33.1).

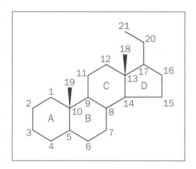

Figure 33.1 The general structure of steroids. Identified are rings A–D and the 21-carbon backbone.

Adrenal steroids

Cortisol/corticosterone

- Species orthologues, where cortisol is the human equivalent of corticosterone, acting at both glucocorticoid and mineralocorticoid receptors.
- Produced in the adrenal cortex zona fasciculata by a cytochrome P450 isoform (CYP11B1, 11β-hydroxylase):
  - introduces a hydroxyl group in the 11-position (converting deoxycorticosterone to corticosterone and 11-deoxycortisol to cortisol; Figure 33.2)
  - loss-of-function mutations are associated with congenital adrenal hyperplasia and hypertension.
- Plasma levels display profound circadian rhythms, where cortisol levels are highest in the subjective morning and lowest during sleep:

Figure 33.2 Synthetic pathways of sex steroids and corticosteroids.

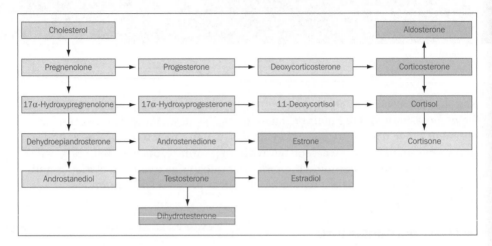

- elevated cortisol levels are associated with increased alertness, but also mood disturbances.

Glucocorticoid receptors (GR)
- Part of the hypothalamic–pituitary–adrenal (HPA) stress response:
  - Glucocorticoids are released at times of stress but there is also a marked diurnal variation, leading to an increase in liver gluconeogenesis and a decrease in peripheral glucose uptake and metabolism, resulting in elevated plasma glucose.
  - GR activation results in a general increase in fat, protein and carbohydrate turnover.
  - Cortisol is much more potent than aldosterone as an agonist.
- An insufficiency of GR activation results in Addisonian crisis (hypotension, shock, death):
  - Insufficient GR activation associated with Addison's disease or pituitary failure is treated by replacement therapy with cortisol.
- Excessive GR activation (often associated with administration of exogenous steroids) results in Cushing's syndrome, 'moon face', osteoporosis, diabetes mellitus, immune suppression, thinning of the skin.
- HPA axis is thought to be overactive in depression.
- GRs are exploited therapeutically in the use of steroidal anti-inflammatories, such as hydrocortisone, prednisolone, beclometasone in the treatment of asthma, inflammatory bowel disease, eczema and hypersensitivity.
- Additionally, glucocorticoids are exploited in the chemotherapy of acute leukaemia and Hodgkin's lymphoma.

Aldosterone
- Aldosterone is a selective agonist of mineralocorticoid receptors.
- Produced in the adrenal cortex zona glomerulosa by a cytochrome P450 (CYP11B2, aldosterone synthase):

- introduces an additional ring (converting corticosterone to aldosterone; Figure 33.2)
- loss-of-function mutations are rare, but may be associated with salt wasting
- a particular single nucleotide polymorphism (C344T) is associated with hypertension
- expression of the aldosterone synthase gene is increased by K^+ ions and angiotensin II-evoked elevations of calcium, leading to elevated circulating levels of aldosterone.
- Plasma aldosterone levels seem to follow a similar diurnal rhythm to cortisol.

Mineralocorticoid receptors (MR)

- Cortisol is equipotent with aldosterone as an agonist; cortisone is very much less effective.
- 11β-hydroxysteroid dehydrogenase, of which two isoforms exist, allows reversible oxidation of 11-hydroxyl to keto group, allowing interconversion of cortisol and cortisone (Figure 33.2):
  - *HSD11B1* is widely distributed and preferentially converts cortisone to the inactive cortisol.
  - In contrast, *HSD11B2* is of limited distribution and appears to be expressed only in those tissues where the mineralocorticoid receptor is expressed and preferentially converts cortisone to cortisol.
  - Mice in which the *hsd11b1* gene is disrupted are less prone to metabolic syndrome, leading to the suggestion that selective inhibitors of this enzyme may have therapeutic potential in this area.
  - In humans, loss-of-function mutations in *HSD11B2* are associated with the syndrome of apparent mineralocorticoid excess (SAME).
- MR have a physiological role in the kidney in the reabsorption of Na^+ in the distal tubule and collecting duct.
- Adrenocortical insufficiency is treated by replacement therapy, usually using a metabolism-resistant analogue, fludrocortisone.
- Oedema associated with liver cirrhosis may be treated by MR antagonists, such as spironolactone and eplerenone, resulting in K^+-sparing diuresis (see Chapter 14).

Gonadal steroids

Testosterone/dihydrotestosterone

- Testosterone is secreted by Leydig cells of the testes.
- It is converted to dihydrotestosterone by 5α-reductase in male skin, seminal vesicles, prostate and epididymus:
  - It reduces a double bond in steroid ring A (Figure 33.2).
  - Gain-of-function mutations of 5α-reductase may prove to be associated with polycystic ovary syndrome.
  - Loss-of-function mutations are associated with intersexualism (cf. hermaphroditism), but are not associated with male-pattern baldness.

- Inhibitors of 5α-reductase include finasteride, used in the treatment of benign prostatic hyperplasia and androgenic alopecia.
- Dihydrotestosterone, unlike testosterone, is not a substrate for aromatase and so represents an irreversible 'male' influence.
- Testosterone supplementation is used as therapy for hypogonadal males and trans-sexual/intersexualism or for the promotion of erythropoiesis in aplastic anaemia.

Androgen receptors (AR)

- Dihydrotestosterone is more potent than testosterone.
- ARs provide for male sexual differentiation in the fetus and development of male sexual characteristics at puberty.
- Amongst the steroid hormone receptors, ARs are the major target for abused drugs, in the exploitation of anabolic steroids among athletes and bodybuilders:
  - Nandrolone, a metabolite of testosterone in naturally low abundance, enhances muscle growth, but has major side-effects ranging from acne to testicular wastage, as well as hepatotoxicity and psychological disturbance.
- AR antagonists (such as cyproterone and flutamide) are used to reduce the progression of some forms of prostate cancer and have also been employed as 'chemical castration'.

Estrone/estradiol

In women of childbearing years, the primary source of gonadal steroids is the ovary.

- Aromatase increases the aromaticity of steroids and converts:
  - androstrenedione to estrone
  - testosterone to estradiol
  - found in ovary, placenta, endometrium, brain, adipose tissue, blood vessels, skin and bone
  - gain-of-function mutations are rare and are associated with gynaecomastia in boys and precocious puberty and gigantomastia in girls
  - loss-of-function mutations have little impact in boys, but are associated with virilisation of girls at birth and primary amenorrhoea.

Oestrogen receptors (ER) and progesterone receptors (PR)

- Responsible for normal female reproductive development and secondary sex characteristics and the regulation of the menstrual cycle, as well as having important roles during pregnancy.

Female contraception

The most common form of contraception ('the pill') typically contains either a progestogen alone (commonly norethisterone, desogestrel, etynodiol or levonorgestrel) or a combination of a synthetic oestrogen (often ethinylestrogen) and a progestogen (often norethisterone, desogestrel, drospirenone or levonorgestrel). The latter formulation is available as a monophasic version with fixed amounts of the component drugs, or as a multiphasic with varying amounts of the two hormones according to the stage of the menstrual cycle.

- The combined oral contraceptive pill exerts its primary effect through inhibition of ovulation.
- The oestrogen component suppresses secretion of the gonadotrophins, luteinising hormone (LH) and follicle-stimulating hormone (FSH), and follicular maturation.
- The progestogen component alters endometrial structure, making embryonic implantation less likely, and also increases the viscosity of cervical mucus, impeding sperm penetration.

Potential issues with the use of female contraceptive pills include cardiovascular risks and sex steroid-dependent cancers, such that past or family history of thromboembolism or hypertension would be possible contraindications. Since progestogens are associated with fewer cardiovascular effects, although the progestogen-only pill shows less clinical efficacy, they may be preferred in those instances.

Hormone replacement therapy (HRT)
- Postmenopause is usually defined as the absence of menstruation for a year, which usually occurs in the mid to late 40s.
- In perimenopausal women, with the exception of the loss of bone density (osteoporosis), the symptoms of cessation of ovarian function vary considerably.
- A frequent symptom identified is hot flashes, although many other symptoms, including mood changes, insomnia, fatigue and memory problems, are also reported.

SERMs
- Expression of ER is elevated in around 70% of breast cancer cases, leading to the use of ER blockers such as tamoxifen and raloxifene.
- Recently the concept of selective nuclear receptor modulators (SNURMs) has developed from the identification of selective oestrogen receptor modulators (SERMs).
- SERMs, such as tamoxifen and raloxifene, are used in the therapy of breast cancer and HRT.
- Effects of SERMS are tissue-specific:
  - tamoxifen – agonist in uterus and bone, but antagonist in breast
  - raloxifene – agonist in bone, antagonist in breast, inactive in uterus.
- This tissue-specific action of SERMs has been suggested to be due to the differential expression of the two subtypes of ER, α and β, or the variation in tissue expression of multiple co-activators for the ER.
- HRT/tamoxifen act as agonists in bone, leading to maintenance of calcium levels and bone strength, and so prevent/reduce osteoporosis in menopausal women.

- These agents have no effect on vasomotor symptoms and exhibit a heightened risk of cardiovascular events (thromboembolism) and uterine cancer.

General principles of steroid hormone receptor activation

- The steroid hormone is lipophilic and readily crosses the plasma membrane to interact with the steroid hormone receptor in the cytosol.
- This receptor is kept quiescent by being attached to a chaperone protein (such as hsp90, a heat shock protein). This is displaced by the steroid hormone and is able to exert biological actions independent of the activated steroid hormone receptors.
- The activated steroid hormone receptors form dimers which migrate to the nucleus, where specialised domains of the receptors interact with particular stretches of DNA, termed a response element, which are located upstream of the target gene.

Figure 33.3 Action of steroid hormone receptors. ER, oestrogen receptor.

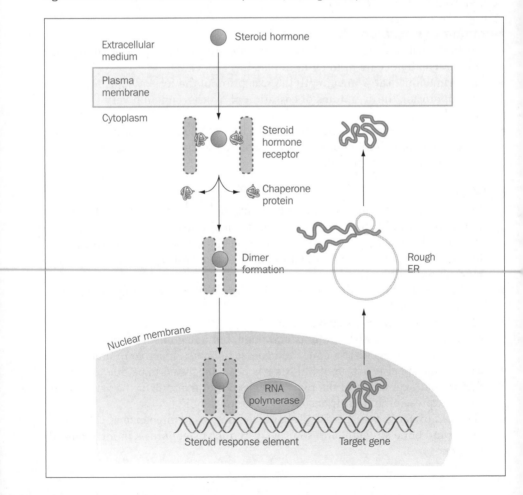

- Under the influence of additional proteins, including co-activators, co-repressors and RNA polymerase (as well as enzymes that regulate histone:DNA interactions), the target gene is transcribed into mRNA, which is exported from the nucleus to the rough endoplasmic reticulum and there translated into protein.
- Overall, this process is slow, with a timescale of many minutes and hours.
- Steroid hormone receptors may be divided into corticosteroid (glucocorticoid and mineralocorticoid) receptors and sex steroid hormone (androgen, oestrogen and progesterone) receptors (Figure 33.3).
- Recently, 7-transmembrane receptors for both oestrogen (GPE) and progestins (mPR) have been identified, although their physiological significance remains to be identified.

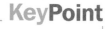

KeyPoint

- Steroids evoke long-lasting responses with a long latency.

Self-assessment

1. **Which of the following is true for adrenal steroid hormones and their receptors?**
a. Aldosterone activates both glucocorticoid and mineralocorticoid receptors.
b. Cortisol is the major endogenous agonist of glucocorticoid receptors in humans.
c. Plasma levels of cortisol are at their peak in the middle of the day.
d. Polymorphisms in the aldosterone synthase gene are associated with hypertension.
e. Steroid therapy in humans can give rise to osteoporosis.

2. **Which of the following is true for gonadal steroid hormones and their receptors?**
a. Tamoxifen may be used to relieve the symptoms of menopause.
b. Progestogens reduce follicular maturation.
c. Aromatase inhibitors increase the accumulation of oestrogens.
d. 5α-reductase inhibitors may be used to reduce the progression of benign prostatic hyperplasia.
e. Testosterone supplementation may be given to stimulate blood cell formation in forms of anaemia.

chapter 34
Biopharmaceuticals

- Biopharmaceuticals are biologically generated drugs, as opposed to the majority of drugs, which are small molecules generated by chemical means. Although many therapeutic agents, from aspirin to paclitaxel, were initially derived from biological sources, they are predominantly generated by large-scale chemical manufacturing methods. In the last decade, the number of new approved biopharmaceutical drugs has remained roughly constant at 2–5 per year. At the same time, the numbers of new small-molecule drugs appear to be slowing from more than 40 per year in the mid-1990s to fewer than 20 in the mid-2000s.
- The majority of biopharmaceuticals are monoclonal antibodies (mAbs), with fewer recombinant hormones, cytokines and clotting factors. Nucleic acids, including antisense oligonucleotides, are also considered as biopharmaceuticals. Although showing promise in preclinical models, only an agent directed at a retinal virus, fomiversen, has reached the clinic. Similarly, gene therapy appears to be an exciting possibility, showing particular promise in the treatment of cystic fibrosis, with as yet unfulfilled potential.
- A feature of the use of biopharmaceuticals is their high cost, which is largely determined by the method of manufacture.

Monoclonal antibodies

Antibodies as therapy
- The major application of mAbs as therapeutic agents is in the treatment of cancers.
- Other therapeutic targets include rheumatoid arthritis and other immune diseases and immunosuppression for organ transplantation.
- Successful therapy for these conditions requires chronic administration.
- Using human spleen/lymph nodes to generate human mAbs has been largely unsuccessful and is ethically questionable.
- Repeated administration in humans of murine antibodies generates an immune response, with the production of human antimouse antibodies.
- One option is to mask or disguise that part of the immunoglobulin G (IgG) molecule that defines 'mouse'.
- Using recombinant techniques it is possible to substitute human Fc regions for rodent Fc (Figure 34.1) to 'humanise' rodent Abs.
- One further alternative is to 'resurface' the rodent Ab, such that amino acids on the exterior of the antibody, which may be recognised as rodent, are replaced with the corresponding amino acids from human IgG.

Figure 34.1 The structure of immunoglobulin G (IgG) antibodies. The Fc is the constant region of the antibody, whereas Fab is the variable region. The antigen recognition domain is also indicated.

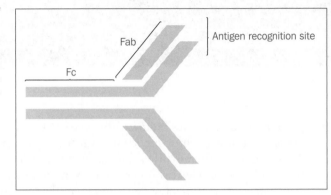

- Two broad approaches have been successfully applied:
  1. In vivo humanised mAbs:
     generate a transgenic mouse where mouse Fc region is replaced with human IgG κ chain
     immunise with antigen
     isolate B cells from spleen/lymph nodes
     screen for Ab-producing cells and clone the cells
     use vat-sized biotechnology to produce pharmaceutically useful amounts of mAb.
  2. In vitro humanised Ab (phage display library):
     The DNA sequences of antibodies are identified as a library from spleen, lymphocytes or bone marrow; they:
     generate human/rodent chimeric antibodies using in vitro recombinant techniques
     insert into bacteriophage genome
     infect *Escherichia coli* and allow it to multiply
     screen for Ab-producing cells and clone
     transfer to mammalian host cell culture since the mAbs are glycoproteins (not synthesised in prokaryotes)
     use vat-sized biotechnology to produce pharmaceutically useful amounts of mAb.
- Examples of monoclonal antibodies in therapeutic use include:
  - omalizumab: IgE antibody for prophylaxis of allergic asthma
  - natalizumab: integrin blocker with mixed success in multiple sclerosis and Crohn's disease
  - rituximab: CD20 blocker with application in non-Hodgkin's lymphoma and rheumatoid arthritis
  - alemtuzumab: CD52 blocker with application in chronic lymphocytic leukaemia and T-cell lymphoma
  - daclizumab: CD25 blocker, preventing high-affinity interleukin-2 binding to lymphocytes, used to prevent transplant rejection.

Recombinant hormones, cytokines and clotting factors

- The major indication for the use of almost all of the recombinant hormone biopharmaceuticals is for the replacement of natural hormones where there is a deficiency.
- Insulin is a good example, where previously extracts of the pancreas from pigs and cattle taken at the abattoir were used for the treatment of diabetes mellitus. With the danger of zootropes – pathogens which may pass across species – the use of animal-derived hormones is in decline, being replaced by biotechnology-generated recombinant proteins.
- Other hormones used as biopharmaceuticals include growth hormone, erythropoietin, follicle-stimulating hormone and colony-stimulating factor.
- Recombinant cytokines, such as interferons α, β and γ and interleukin-2, may be used in the treatment of some cancers or long-term immune disorders, such as multiple sclerosis.
  - There are two biopharmaceutical approaches to reducing the effectiveness of elevated inflammatory cytokine levels.
  - The interleukin-1 receptor antagonist is a large protein, which can be synthesised in vitro using recombinant techniques. It is used in the treatment of rheumatoid arthritis.
  - Etanercept is a fusion protein, which is made up of a portion of the soluble receptor for tumour necrosis factor (TNF-α) linked to the Fc region of IgG. Infusion reduces circulating levels of tumour necrosis factor-α, leading to relief of some of the symptoms of rheumatoid arthritis and severe psoriasis.
- Numerous proteins are involved in the clotting process (see Chapter 15); biopharmaceuticals have therapeutic uses in this area:
  - Clotting factors include recombinant factor VIII and factor IX, used in the treatment of haemophilias.
  - Tissue plasminogen activator, generated as a recombinant protein, is used for thrombolysis in the acute treatment of stroke, pulmonary embolism and myocardial infarction.

KeyPoint

- Biopharmaceuticals are an expensive group of drugs, with applications primarily in the areas of cancer and immunotherapy.

The general public are aware that sometimes the effectiveness of drugs can wear off with continued usage or sometimes the drugs just don't work. There may be many reasons for this, not least of all misdiagnosis of the disease/disorder. One common reason for a lack of clinical efficacy is poor patient compliance. This is typified by the failure to complete a course of antibiotics, which, despite an initial improvement in symptoms, can fail to eradicate completely the underlying bacterial infection, resulting in a recurrence of the infection. Lack of adherence to the prescribed regimen of antibiotics can have more serious implications for the whole population as it is also associated with development of antibiotic resistance, another cause of reduced clinical efficacy.

Tachyphylaxis

- Desensitisation and tachyphylaxis: repeated or continuous application of agonist over a timescale of minutes results in a reduced responsiveness to the agonist.
- Tolerance is the same phenomenon: a much slower decline in responsiveness, generally considered to occur within days or weeks.
- Mechanisms involved in receptor desensitisation may be one or several of the following:
  - changes in receptor–effector coupling: these effects are rapid – for transmitter-gated channels, this can occur in fractions of seconds
  - changes in receptor number
  - exhaustion of mediators: for example, amphetamine depletes stores of releasable noradrenaline and so repeated applications show decreased responsiveness
  - increased effects or induction of drug catabolism, for example, nicotine induces a particular isoform of cytochrome P450, which is also responsible for metabolism of the antipsychotic clozapine
  - physiological adaptation: the effect is nullified by normal physiological homoeostatic mechanisms.

Receptor desensitisation

- The receptor, which has been most investigated in terms of mechanisms of desensitisation, is probably the β_2-adrenoceptor (β_2AR). Desensitisation of the β_2AR is evoked in three identifiable steps.
- The most rapid step in β_2AR desensitisation is uncoupling of the receptor from the G-protein. This involves a rapid reduction of receptor-stimulated

cyclic adenosine monophosphate (cAMP) generation (a reduced functional response) and a loss in guanosine triphosphate (GTP)-sensitive, high-affinity agonist binding (a modified receptor–G-protein interaction):

- There are two mechanisms involved in G-protein uncoupling, both of which entail receptor phosphorylation.
- Elevated levels of intracellular cAMP evoked by agonist activation of the receptor lead to protein kinase A-dependent phosphorylation of serine residues on the β_2AR at one of two sites: on the third intracellular loop or on the cytoplasmic carboxy terminal. This pathway completes a negative-feedback loop, by introducing dense negative charges into the regions of the receptor which couple to the G-protein.
- G$\beta\gamma$ subunits of the G-protein can activate a G-protein-coupled receptor kinase (GRK), of which one isoform is β-adrenoceptor kinase (βARK). βARK can phosphorylate multiple serine and threonine residues on the cytoplasmic carboxy terminal of the β_2AR. This phosphorylation alone is insufficient to uncouple the receptor from the G-protein, but it allows recruitment and reversible attachment of a subsidiary protein, β-arrestin, which effectively blocks access of the G-protein to the β_2AR.
- The timescale of these events is relatively rapid, with interruption of G-protein coupling observable within less than 5 min, with the protein kinase A route being more prevalent at lower agonist concentrations, and the βARK pathway active at higher agonist concentrations.

■ The second mechanism of receptor desensitisation involves internalisation of the receptor.

- After longer agonist exposure, receptors are found in intracellular compartments, termed endosomes.
- Uncoupled receptors are internalised (sequestered) away from the cell surface through β-arrestin interaction with clathrin (coated pit formation).
- This appears to be primarily a mechanism for receptor recycling, as the endosomes undergo acidification, which induces a conformational change in the phosphorylated receptor, allowing it to be dephosphorylated by a protein phosphatase (PP2A). The receptor may then be reinserted into the plasma membrane by a mechanism that is as yet undefined.

■ The third and slowest step in receptor desensitisation is downregulation. This is a complete disappearance of receptors, with a loss in total cellular binding, and involves degradation of the receptor. It can only be reversed by de novo receptor protein synthesis.

- Endosomes containing internalised receptors can sort receptors to lysosomes for proteolytic degradation.
- Parallel mechanisms exist which are as yet incompletely defined, but which appear not to require receptor internalisation.
- Concurrent with increased receptor degradation is a reduced receptor synthesis, which is mediated through a genomic action of protein kinase A acting on nuclear transcription factors to repress β_2AR gene transcription.

- At the same time as β_2AR downregulation, other components of the signalling cascade may also be altered. For example, the G-protein may be downregulated, while phosphodiesterase levels may increase.
■ Although these mechanisms appear to hold true for β_2ARs, it is apparent that they represent a useful model, but are not universally applicable. Indeed, these mechanisms can vary not only between different receptors, but also between different cell types.

Tolerance to heroin

Repeated administration of heroin results in:
■ reduced euphoric effect
■ reduced respiratory effects
■ maintained effect on constipation and pupil constriction.
the effects of heroin are mediated primarily through activation of mu (μ) opioid peptide (MOP) receptors, which can be phosphorylated by βARK; the phosphorylated MOP receptor can bind β-arrestin; the MOP receptor internalises and downregulates.
■ This is true for the high-efficacy agonists DAMGO and fentanyl, but not the partial agonist morphine.
■ Tolerance to morphine can be explained by three mechanisms, which may act independently or in combination:
   1. Changes in signal transduction partners other than the receptor. Certain isoforms of adenylyl cyclase are increased following protracted exposure to morphine, reverting cellular cAMP levels back to normal.
   2. Changes in functionally antagonistic transmitters. At the spinal cord level, cholecystokinin (CCK) reduces the analgesic effect of morphine. Release of antiopioid peptides (including CCK) increases in morphine tolerance and these antiopioid peptides may contribute to withdrawal symptoms on discontinuation of heroin.
   3. Changes in neural networks. MOP receptors are expressed on an intermediate neurone in a series. Acute exposure to morphine reduces activity of the intermediate neurone, thereby reducing the activity of the network overall. During prolonged exposure to morphine, the downstream neurones compensate in some way for the reduced input from the MOP-expressing neurone and the overall output from the network is normalised once more.

Receptor desensitisation and downregulation may be clinically useful

There are examples when receptor desensitisation or downregulation may be desirable:
■ Downregulation of β-adrenoceptors in the central nervous system correlates with the beneficial effects of antidepressants (see Chapter 20). One version of the monoamine theory of depression, which postulates underactivity of monoamine neurotransmission, suggests that downregulation of β-adrenoceptors allows normalisation of neurotransmitter–receptor interactions.

- Gonadotrophin-releasing hormone (GnRH) receptor agonists, such as goserelin, are used in the treatment of hormone-sensitive cancers, principally of the prostate and breast (see Chapter 32). The heightened potency of the synthetic agonists accelerates desensitisation and downregulation of hypothalamic GnRH receptors, leading to a reduction in circulating gonadal steroid hormones and reduced progression of the cancers.
- Capsaicin is used as a topical treatment for neuropathic and musculoskeletal pain. It causes a rapid and profound activation of TRPV1 vanilloid receptors on primary afferent neurones, leading to a rapid desensitisation. Subjectively, the transient activation of TRPV1 receptors appears as a burning sensation, which precedes the analgesia. The burning sensation may be sufficiently intense that the patient prefers other medication.

Receptor upregulation

- Long-term treatment with receptor antagonists can lead to the phenomenon of receptor upregulation. For example, after withdrawal from chronic propranolol (β-AR antagonist), 'rebound' tachycardia and increased angina may be observed for up to 3–4 days.
- Hypersensitivity to infusions of catecholamines is also evident after propranolol withdrawal.
- In lymphocytes from these patients, an increased β-AR number on lymphocytes is observed, which returns to baseline levels after several days.

The pharmacodynamic basis of interindividual variation

- If the drug is an inhibitor/antagonist, the level of natural substrate/agonist determines whether the drug has an effect.
- If the drug is an agonist, the level of natural substrate/agonist determines whether the drug has an effect.

Variation in target density
- Cells respond to changes in local external and internal environment by altering expression of proteins (plasticity).
- The previous drug or disease history of the patient can influence the response to drugs by altering the expression level of the target protein.

Variation in target sequence
- Most proteins have some genetic variation:
  - For example, haemoglobin is a heterotetramer ($\alpha_2\beta_2$), where the α_1 isoform (*HBA1*) has 349 variants, the α_2 isoform (*HBA2*) has 293 variants and the β isoform (*HBB*) has 401 variants.
- Many drug targets have identified small genetic variations (single nucleotide polymorphisms: SNPs), which change:
  - levels of protein expression
  - responses to ligands.

- Of the 83 reported SNPs of the β_2-adrenoceptor, the nucleotide shift 46G→A results in a protein change of 16R→G (arginine to glycine, in about 40% of the population).
  - Patients homozygous for Arg16 show greater responses to oral β-agonists and an increased desensitisation to infused isoprenaline.
  - Patients homozygous for Gly16, however, are less responsive, but show no significant wane in responsiveness.
  - Gly16 expression is also associated with nocturnal asthma.

KeyPoint

- Long-term drug administration can lead to reduced clinical efficacy, which may be mediated through multiple mechanisms.

Answers to self-tests

Chapter 4
1. c Omeprazole inhibits H^+/K^+-ATPase activity in the gastric parietal cell, thereby reducing gastric acid output.
2. a AZT is a substrate for nucleoside transporters, thereby allowing access to the reverse transcriptase associated with human immunodeficiency virus (HIV).
3. ATP activates SERCA (b), Na^+/K^+-ATPase (d) and CFTR (e).
4. Both IP_3 (c) and ryanodine receptors (d) can be activated by calcium ions, albeit at different concentrations. Micromolar calcium ion concentrations can activate IP_3 receptors, while millimolar levels inhibit them and activate ryanodine receptors.

Chapter 6
1. a The neurotransmitter released by all preganglionic autonomic neurones is *acetylcholine.*
    b The receptors for ACh on all postganglionic autonomic neurones are of the *nicotinic* type.
    c *Noradrenaline* is the neurotransmitter released by most postganglionic sympathetic neurones.
    d The receptors for ACh on most tissues innervated by the parasympathetic system are of the *muscarinic* type.
2. a True.
    b False; there are many NANC transmitters such as nitric oxide, VIP, ATP.
    c False; they are co-transmitters in the sympathetic system.
    d False; monoamine oxidase controls intracellular noradrenaline levels. The action of released noradrenaline is terminated by reuptake.
3. a Blood vessels have very little *parasympathetic* innervation.
    b Gut motility is increased by activation of the *parasympathetic* division of the ANS.
    c Bronchial smooth muscle is relaxed by *noradrenaline* and contracted by *acetylcholine* (other answers are possible – suggest some!).
    d Blockade of muscarinic receptors in the pupillary smooth muscle causes *dilatation* of the pupil.
4. a, d
5. a Prazosin is a selective antagonist of a_1-*adrenoceptors.*
    b Ephedrine is an *indirectly acting* sympathomimetic drug,
    c a_1-adrenoceptors are linked to the $G_{q/11}$ *protein* and cause Ca^{2+} mobilisation.
    d $β_2$-adrenoceptor agonists (e.g. salbutamol) are used in the treatment of *asthma (or COPD)* because they cause *bronchodilatation.*

Chapter 7

1. Nitric oxide is generated by the enzyme nitric oxide *synthase*.
2. Nitric oxide activates the enzyme *soluble* guanylyl cyclase.
3. Arachidonic acid is found in the *C-2* position of most membrane phospholipids.
4. Cytochrome P450-like enzymes metabolise arachidonic acid to form *epoxyeicosatrienoic acids*.
5. 5-Lipoxygenase activity can be inhibited by *protein kinase A*.
6. Leukotriene A_4 is generated by *5-lipoxygenase* activity.
7. Montelukast blocks *CysLT$_1$* receptors.
8. LXA_4 is a full agonist at *ALX* LX receptors.
9. COX activity converts arachidonic acid to *prostaglandin H_2*.
10. PGs are inactivated by the enzyme *15-hydroxyprostaglandin dehydrogenase*.

Chapter 8

1. True.
2. False; it is volume per time.
3. True.
4. False; it means that 5% is eliminated per day.
5. True; $\log_e 2/k = 0.693/0.05 = 13.9$ h.

Chapter 9

1. a True.
   b False, because triple therapy is the combination of two antibiotics and usually a PPI.
   c False, because COX-1 inhibition is regarded as the important target.
   d False, because misoprostol is actually cytoprotective.
2. d PPIs reduce acid secretion. H_1 antagonists are used for allergy and do not affect H_2 receptors in the stomach; agents that increase cAMP are linked to acid secretion; gastrin is the physiological stimulus.

Chapter 10

1. a and d. Antibiotics and orlistat are associated with diarrhoea due to superinfection and steatorrhoea respectively.
2. b and c. Opioids and muscarinic antagonists lead to constipation via presynaptic and postsynaptic inhibition respectively.

Chapter 11

4 and 5 are antiemetics. 3 and 6 are associated with causing nausea.

Chapter 12

1. a True.
   b True.
   c True.
   d False: digoxin reduces AVN conduction.
   e False: it may enhance entry or decrease efflux.

2. a (calcium channel antagonists) and d (digoxin) reduce heart rate.
   b Dihydropyridines do not affect cardiac cells. c Antimuscarinic agents
   block vagal control and will increase heart rate. e β-adrenoceptor agonists
   will stimulate cardiac β_1-adrenoceptors and increase heart rate.

Chapter 13

1. c ACEIs should not be used in renovascular disease as this may cause
   severe hypotension and renal damage. They are used in CHF and
   hypokalaemia is not a problem. They can be used safely in asthma but, if
   an ACEI-induced cough develops, this could pose a problem.
2. d Asthma is a contraindication to β-blockers due to the risk of
   bronchoconstriction.
3. c The reduction in heart rate allows more time for coronary flow, which
   only occurs during diastole. β-blockers do not cause coronary
   vasodilatation.
4. a Verapamil will decrease the heart rate. b, c and d will all result from
   calcium channel blockade.
5. c The sodium pump is the target.

Chapter 14

1. a (loop diuretics) and b (thiazides) cause K^+ loss; c and do not.
   c (mineralocorticoid antagonists) are K^+-sparing.
   d (ACE inhibitors) are not diuretics but can cause hyperkalaemia.
2. a False; thiazides inhibit an NaCl transporter.
   b False; loop diuretics inhibit an $Na^+/2Cl^-/K^+$ symporter,
   c True.
   d False; mineralocorticoid receptor antagonists do not affect renin.
3. They are all true.

Chapter 15

1. a
2. f
3. b
4. d
5. a
6. f
7. c

Chapter 17

1. All may be involved except c (adrenaline), which is associated with
   bronchodilation.
2. d (simulation of β_2-adrenoceptors coupled to an increase in cAMP) is the
   mode of action. a There is no anti-inflammatory action. b There is no
   involvement of potassium channels. c They do not block the actions of
   adrenaline.

3. a True, due to an interaction preventing the breakdown of cAMP.
   b False, β_2-agonists and/or muscarinic antagonists are first choice in COPD.
   c True.
   d False, they are phosphodiesterase inhibitors.
4. All except a (corticosteroids) may provoke attacks in certain patients.

Chapter 18
1. False; histamine H_2 receptor antagonists are used in dyspepsia.
2. False; newer agents are not usually associated with sedation.
3. True.
4. True.

Chapter 19
1. True; benzodiazepines are used for both.
2. False; they allosterically increase GABA binding.
3. False; nitrazepam is longer-acting.
4. False; short-acting benzodiazepines have greater potential to cause dependence.
5. True; although benzodiazepines have sedative effects they can paradoxically cause unexpected aggression.
6. False; it is a $5HT_{1A}$ partial agonist.
7. True.
8. False; the β-adrenoceptor antagonist oxprenolol can attenuate the somatic symptoms of anxiety but has no effect on the psychological components.
9. False; anxiolytic drugs are counterproductive if used alone to treat depression, despite anxiety being a common component of major depression. Some antidepressants are licensed to treat generalised anxiety disorder (e.g. paroxetine) so these would be a compelling choice for depression with a significant anxiety component.
10. False; barbiturates are highly toxic, have great abuse potential, cause dependence and have no place in anxiety therapy apart from treating intractable insomnia in patients already stabilised on a barbiturate.

Chapter 20
1. a, c, d Citalopram is a selective reuptake inhibitor, venlafaxine is an SNRI (it inhibits both noradrenaline and 5HT reuptake) and the components of St John's wort have a combination of properties, including inhibition of monoamine reuptake and MAO. Reboxetine is a noradrenaline reuptake inhibitor.
2. c Lithium and carbamazepine are of use prophylactically but if acute antimanic action is required, the neuroleptic prochlorperazine is effective.
3. a (possibly!) Given the fact that most antidepressants increase synaptic monoamine availability, the monoamine hypothesis probably has some truth, but cocaine and amphetamine also increase monoamine availability and are not antidepressant and tianeptine is effective despite reducing 5HT availability. No

class of antidepressant is more effective than any other, overall, but individual patients can benefit from switching drugs. Because they have long half-lives a washout period of 1–2 weeks is required when switching.

4. a, c, d   Blockade of muscarinic acetylcholine receptors produces urinary retention and constipation. Cardiotoxicity, as shown by electrocardiographic abnormalities, can be fatal. Suicidal patients should not have access to such toxic drugs.

5. a, b, d   MAOIs potentiate the actions of the sympathomimetic (act like noradrenaline) agents such as tyramine, found in mature cheese (also beef and yeast extracts, pickled herrings, Chianti and other red wines) and decongestants (e.g. ephedrine, xylometazoline). Potentiation of the effects of TCAs could lead to fatal hypertension.

Chapter 21

1. a   A *partial* seizure has a focal starting point in the brain.
   b   A *generalised* seizure has no focal point and begins in both cerebral hemispheres.
   c   An *absence* seizure involves brief lapses of consciousness.
   d   A *tonic/clonic (grand mal)* seizure is generalised and involves stiffening or rigidity of the entire body followed by rhythmic movements of the limbs.

2. a   *Ethosuximide* or *valproate* is first-line therapy for absence seizures.
   b   *Valproate* is first-line therapy for myoclonic seizures.
   c   *Carbamazepine, lamotrigine, topiramate* or *oxcarbazepine* is first-line therapy for partial seizures.
   d   *Carbamazepine, lamotrigine, topiramate* or *valproate* is first-line therapy for grand mal seizures.

3. a   True,
   b   True; it also blocks voltage-activated Ca^{2+} channels.
   c   False; it blocks T-type Ca^{2+} channels.
   d   True; it activates the benzodiazepine allosteric binding site on the $GABA_A$ receptor, increasing its affinity for GABA.

4. b and d are true.
   a   Phenytoin can cause gingival hyperplasia, acne and hirsutism.
   c   Medicated patients suffering from epilepsy are, however, allowed to drive a private motor vehicle providing they have been seizure-free for 1 year or if they have only suffered seizures during sleep for a period of 3 years.

Chapter 22

1. a   Antipsychotic drugs are also known as major tranquillisers and *neuroleptics*.
   b   All antipsychotics are antagonists of *dopamine D_2* receptors.
   c   If two other antipsychotics have proved to be ineffective, *clozapine* should be prescribed.
   d   The movement disorder side-effect of *tardive dyskinesia* can appear months after the start of antipsychotic therapy.

2. a and c. Antipsychotics can cause parkinsonian tremor and should be used with great caution in the elderly, particularly if there is a history of stroke.
3. a True; so is risperidone.
    b False; akathisia (restlessness) is an antipsychotic side-effect.
    c False; intramuscular doses should be lower as they avoid first-pass metabolism.
    d True.

Chapter 23

1. a (bradykinesia) and b (muscle tremor) are characteristic but c (depression) and d (dementia) are commonly associated with PD.
2. The ergot derivatives a (bromocriptine) and b (pergolide).
3. The peripheral COMT inhibitor b (tolcapone) and the peripheral dopa-decarboxylase inhibitor d (carbidopa). The monoamine oxidase inhibitor-B c (selegiline) enhances dopamine survival in the brain.
4. According to the National Institute for Health and Clinical Excellence, there is no single drug of choice in early-stage PD treatment. Given the movement disorder side-effects of levodopa, first choice would probably be b (rotigotine: dopamine receptor agonist), before initiating a (levodopa) along with enzyme inhibitors.

Chapter 24

1. a Nausea is common. Opioids are associated with constipation, pupillary constriction and postural hypotension.
2. b Pethidine has a rapid onset, relatively brief period of action and is not very constipating.
3. a Paracetamol is often mistakenly classed as an NSAID but has little or no anti-inflammatory actions.
4. c (neuropathic pain) and d (trigeminal neuralgia). Gabapentin is most often used for neuropathic pain.
5. b (gastric ulcer), c (heart failure) and d (asthma).

Chapter 25

1. c (nicotine). The others have minor risks of causing true dependence when used at usual doses.
2. b Intravenous administration delivers the largest bolus dose to the brain, producing the most intense effects. Nasal and buccal absorption is also rapid and is a common means of administration. Inhalation (cocaine, heroin, tobacco) also provides rapid drug delivery and is a favoured route.
3. c Naltrexone is a pure opioid receptor antagonist and blocks effects of all opioid agonists, including heroin. It is used to counteract overdose but will precipitate a withdrawal syndrome in regular users. Buprenorphine is a partial opioid receptor agonist so will reduce the effects of efficacious agonists such as heroin and is used in substitution therapy. Methadone is

a partial agonist but its half-life is much longer, reducing the craving that follows the rapid increase and decrease in circulating heroin levels after intravenous administration. Benzodiazepines like temazepam actually increase the intensity of heroin's effects when taken together but they can be helpful in reducing withdrawal symptoms.

4. a, c, d. Disulfiram has unpleasant interactions with alcohol and (in theory) discourages drinking. Acamprosate reduces withdrawal symptoms. Clomethiazole, is a helpful sedative and also inhibits alcohol dehydrogenase, which slows the rate of alcohol elimination and reduces withdrawal symptoms. Buproprion has some value in treating smoking cessation craving.

5. a Many patients became dependent upon prescription benzodiazepines such as temazepam used as anxiolytics; the prolonged withdrawal symptoms may be worse.

Chapter 26

1. a False: mechanisms are unclear but there may be differing targets according to the particular agent.
    b True.
    c True.
    d False: some are analgesic (e.g. ketamine) and others are not (e.g. thiopental).
    e False: this is true of gaseous agents.

Chapter 27

1. b, d.
2. b, c

Chapter 28

1. False: they do not affect levels of T_4 and T_3.
2. True: there is a significant adverse effect.
3. True: hence the use of β-blockers for symptomatic relief.
4. False: the long half-life of thyroid hormones means that a response is delayed.
5. False: T_3 is the more active form and this acts via nuclear thyroid hormone receptors.

Chapter 29

1. c (glucose via ATP), d (sulphonylureas) and e (exenatide) all evoke insulin release. Metformin does not and it is cell depolarisation, not hyperpolarisation, that causes release.
2. a (insulin) and c (sulphonylureas) may be associated with hypoglycaemia; b (metformin) and d (acarbose) are not.
3. Insulin, b; metformin, d; sulphonylureas, e; thiazolidiniediones, a.

Chapter 30

1. b (amoxicillin) and d (vancomycin). Erythromycin and chloramphenicol interfere with bacterial protein synthesis and ciprofloxacin is a bacterial DNA gyrase inhibitor.
2. a (erythromycin) with 4 (drug interactions due to enzyme inhibition); b (amoxicillin) with 5 (destruction by β-lactamase); c (chloramphenicol (oral)) with 2 (aplastic anaemia); d (rifampicin) with 3 (drug interactions due to enzyme induction); e (gentamicin) with 1 (ototoxicity).

Chapter 31

1. (aciclovir) with d (inhibits viral DNA polymerase) and g (herpes)
2. (zanamivir) with c (neuramidase inhibitor) and i (influenza)
3. (zidovudine) with e (nucleoside reverse transcriptase inhibitor) and h (anti-HIV)
4. (clotrimazole) with b (inhibits conversion of lanosterol to ergosterol) and j (antifungal)
5. (proguanil) with a (folate antagonist) and f (antimalarial)

Chapter 32

1. Particular alleles of the *BRCA1* gene predispose to *breast and ovarian* cancer.
2. *Helicobacter pylori* infection is associated with an elevated risk of gastric cancer.
3. Methotrexate inhibits the enzyme *dihydrofolate reductase*.
4. Cyclophosphamide action can be diverted in tissues expressing high activities of the enzyme *aldehyde dehydrogenase*.
5. Etoposide, a podophyllotoxin, inhibits activity of the enzyme *topoisomerase*.
6. Vincristine inhibits *microtubule* function.
7. Tamoxifen is used to treat breast cancers by blocking *oestrogen* receptors.
8. *Trastuzumab* is a monoclonal antibody which targets one of the subunits of the EGF receptor in the treatment of some breast cancers.
9. The Philadelphia chromosome is a translocation of chromosomes, and is associated with *chronic myeloid* leukaemia.
10. A major cause of drug resistance is an increased expression of the P-*glycoprotein, multidrug resistance protein 1, ABCA2* transporter.

Chapter 33

1. a False; aldosterone activates mineralocorticoid receptors selectively.
   b True.
   c False; plasma levels of cortisol are at their peak in the morning.
   d True.
   e True.

2. a True.
   b True.
   c False; aromatase inhibitors increase the accumulation of testosterone and
      decrease the production of oestrogens.
   d True.
   e True, particularly in aplastic anaemia.

Index

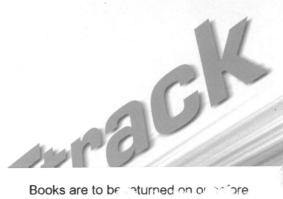

Books are to be returned on or before

Pharmacology